ECG Interpretation for Everyone

ECG Interpretation for Everyone
An On-The-Spot Guide

Fred Kusumoto MD
Associate Professor of Medicine
Director of Electrophysiology and Pacing
Division of Cardiovascular Diseases
Department of Medicine
Mayo Clinic
Jacksonville, FL, USA

Pam Bernath RN, RN-C
Division of Cardiovascular Diseases
Department of Medicine
Mayo Clinic
Jacksonville, FL, USA

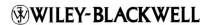

A John Wiley & Sons, Ltd., Publication

To Dr. Edward H. Wyman
and to Laura, Miya, Hana, and Aya

Registered Office
John Wiley & Sons, Ltd, The Atrium, Southern Gate, Chichester, West Sussex, PO19 8SQ, UK

Editorial Offices
9600 Garsington Road, Oxford, OX4 2DQ, UK
The Atrium, Southern Gate, Chichester, West Sussex, PO19 8SQ, UK
111 River Street, Hoboken, NJ 07030-5774, USA

For details of our global editorial offices, for customer services and for information about how to apply for permission to reuse the copyright material in this book please see our website at www.wiley.com/wiley-blackwell

Library of Congress Cataloging-in-Publication Data

Kusumoto, Fred.
ECG interpretation for everyone : an on-the-spot guide / Fred Kusumoto and Pam Bernath.
    p. ; cm.
  Includes bibliographical references and index.
  ISBN-13: 978-0-470-65556-6 (pbk. : alk. paper)
  ISBN-10: 0-470-65556-9
I. Bernath, Pam. II. Title. [DNLM: 1. Electrocardiography–Atlases. 2. Electrocardiography–Handbooks. WG 39] LC classification not assigned
  616.1'207547–dc23

                                    2011030261

A catalogue record for this book is available from the British Library.

Wiley also publishes its books in a variety of electronic formats. Some content that appears in print may not be available in electronic books.

Set in 8/11pt Frutiger by SPi Publisher Services, Pondicherry, India

1   2012

Contents

Master Algorithm

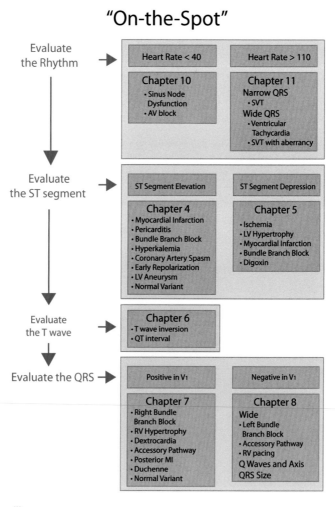

"On-the-Spot"

Evaluate the Rhythm

Heart Rate < 40	Heart Rate > 110
Chapter 10 • Sinus Node Dysfunction • AV block	**Chapter 11** Narrow QRS • SVT Wide QRS • Ventricular Tachycardia • SVT with aberrancy

Evaluate the ST segment

ST Segment Elevation	ST Segment Depression
Chapter 4 • Myocardial Infarction • Pericarditis • Bundle Branch Block • Hyperkalemia • Coronary Artery Spasm • Early Repolarization • LV Aneurysm • Normal Variant	**Chapter 5** • Ischemia • LV Hypertrophy • Myocardial Infarction • Bundle Branch Block • Digoxin

Evaluate the T wave

Chapter 6   • T wave inversion   • QT interval

Evaluate the QRS

Positive in V1	Negative in V1
Chapter 7 • Right Bundle Branch Block • RV Hypertrophy • Dextrocardia • Accessory Pathway • Posterior MI • Duchenne • Normal Variant	**Chapter 8** Wide • Left Bundle Branch Block • Accessory Pathway • RV pacing Q Waves and Axis QRS Size

Preface

I have always been fascinated with learning more about the ECG, and over the last eight years, I have felt a growing desire to learn more about ECG interpretation. I feel that it is an essential tool that should be used on a regular basis by medical personnel who care for patients. After countless hours of study and the awareness that most people do not have this much time to spend on this subject, I realized the need for a "quick reference ECG recognition guide." ECG changes can happen quickly and decisions will need to be made "on the spot". This book is intended for this purpose because it can help the interpreter recognize key elements on the ECG that are pertinent to different arrhythmias or conditions. The book covers multiple ECGs with short descriptions of the arrhythmias or conditions, the ECG changes that can occur, and the clinical importance of each ECG change. The medical staff and physicians that work in any monitored unit, especially the emergency rooms and ICUs, should become more familiar with arrhythmias or changes that could represent ischemia, infarction, or dangerous cardiac arrhythmias. Hopefully, this handy pocket ECG guide will help make ECG identification more commonplace.

I would like to thank the nurses in the stress testing department and the ECG technicians at the Mayo Clinic. My two daughters, Alisa and Haley, and other family members have been with me through the long hours of being isolated in my office and they have supported and encouraged me during this busy time. Without the loving support of my husband, Mike, I would never have been able to start or complete this project. I would also like to thank my stepfather and mother, Dr. and Mrs. Edward H. Wyman, for encouraging me when they realized that I had a passion for ECG interpretation in my early years of nursing.

Pam Bernath, RN, RN-C

Pam Bernath is the major force behind this project that is designed to provide an introduction to ECG interpretation. She identified an unmet need for a simple text that would provide the basics of ECG interpretation for the many different healthcare providers that use the ECG on a frequent basis. In thinking about the format of this book we were drawn to the idea of providing an illustration oriented "field guide" for rapid evaluation of ECGs. As a child I still remember pouring over Zim's Guide to Butterflies and Moths (Golden Books, New York). I still have my well-worn friend that accompanied me on afternoon and weekend day trips to the country fields behind my house. After a short introduction, the book covered each of the major butterfly families using drawings, maps, and short paragraphs. This book is designed in a similar manner with a short introduction followed by ECG examples and important "keys" that help identify the critical diagnostic points. I hope that this small pocket book will help you identify ECGs as you are "out in the field," just as Herbert Zim taught me the basics about butterflies and moths.

I too would like to thank my family for putting up with lost weekends and a somewhat distracted husband and dad. Finally, thank you to Sumiko and Howard Kusumoto who encouraged a naturally inquisitive son to look even more closely at the world around him.

Fred Kusumoto, MD

CHAPTER 1

Technical Issues

It is always a bit worrisome when the first chapter has such a dry and uninspiring title, but it is extremely important to understand the fundamentals of the electrocardiogram (ECG) before using the ECG as a clinical tool. The ECG was originally developed over a century ago by Willem Einthoven and has become one of the most important diagnostic tools used for evaluating the heart. Very simply, the heart can be compared to a pump with a primary function of transporting blood to different parts of the body. "Control" of the pump requires an electrical system and, in the heart, contraction of the chambers begins and is controlled by electrical currents generated by cells with spontaneous electrical activity (also called pacemaker activity). The electrical activity produced by the heart causes small electrical changes on the skin that can be measured using skin electrodes. Don't worry; with an average voltage of 1 mV or less, your body won't power a flashlight. The electrodes are connected to a recording machine with special electronics that amplify and enhance the signal. In one subspecialty field of cardiology called electrophysiology, instead of measuring electrical activity from the body surface, electrical activity is measured directly from the inside of the heart chambers using specialized catheters, that are essentially wires coated with insulation and a metal electrode at the tip, inserted into one of the vessels of the body and threaded to the heart itself.

Before we can talk about the ECG and the heart, we have to discuss some extremely dry concepts that describe some of the technical issues on how the ECG is obtained. Although this portion of the book can be extremely mundane, details about electrodes, leads, and the ECG display are important and form the basis for understanding the ECG. Perhaps suffer through this first chapter with only a cursory read and come back to this chapter after you have read some of the other portions of the book.

ECG Interpretation for Everyone: An On-The-Spot Guide, First Edition.
Fred Kusumoto and Pam Bernath.
© 2012 John Wiley & Sons, Ltd. Published 2012 by John Wiley & Sons, Ltd.

Electrode placement

The ECG uses electrodes placed on the skin to measure the cardiac electrical activity. Obtaining good quality images is essential for proper interpretation and requires good and stable contact between the electrode and the skin. As an interesting aside, one of the seminal figures of cardiology, Augustus Waller (who provided the first comprehensive discussion of electrical activity of the heart), used a mouth electrode as a standard position, probably because this surface allowed better conductivity of electrical signals. In the past, to improve electrical conductivity, specialized gel was used between the skin and the metal electrodes. Now almost universally in industrialized nations, the electrodes are small specially designed disposable patches that have a light adhesive that also acts as a conductor to optimize transmission of the electrical signal from the skin to the ECG machine. Generally, the ECG is recorded while the patient is lying on his or her back (supine position) to avoid artifact introduced from body movement. Sometimes patient conditions such as tremors (Parkinson's disease) or interference from other electrical equipment may make recording an ECG difficult. Within the ECG machine itself are special electronics that amplify the electrical signal and filter the electrical signal to "clean-up" the recording. As will be described later, sometimes the ECG is recorded while the patient is exercising on a treadmill. In order to reduce the artifact, these specialized machines use additional electronic circuitry to remove the excess noise introduced by body motion.

To obtain a 12 lead ECG, 10 electrodes are placed on the extremities and the chest (Figure 1.1). One electrode is placed on each of the four extremities: left and right arms and left and right legs. The extremities can be compared to "extension cords" and the ECG signal will not be affected by the exact position of the electrode on the extremity. In contrast, placing a limb electrode on the trunk will lead to some changes in the signals recorded by the ECG. The remaining six electrodes are placed on the anterior chest in specific positions. Collectively the chest electrodes are often called the precordial (the word comes from Latin – *prae*, "front of," and *cor*, "heart") leads and usually referred to as V_1 through V_6 moving from right to left on the chest. The V_1 electrode is placed in the fourth intercostal space just to the right of the sternum and the V_2 electrode is placed in the fourth intercostal space just to the left of the sternum. The V_4 electrode is placed in the fifth intercostal space in

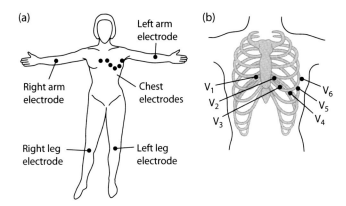

Figure 1.1:

(a): The location for the standard 10 electrodes used to record a 12 lead ECG.

(b): A close-up for the exact positions of the six chest electrodes.

See the text for specific description. (Reproduced with permission from FM Kusumoto, *Cardiovascular Pathophysiology*, Hayes Barton Press, Raleigh, NC, 2004.)

line with the middle of the clavicle (collar bone). The V_3 electrode is placed half way between V_2 and V_4. The V_5 electrode is also placed in the fifth intercostal space at the same level as the V_4 electrode but is located on the left anterior axillary line. The left anterior axillary line is an imaginary vertical line that extends from the front crease of the armpit (*axilla* is the Latin word for "armpit" or "side"). The V_6 electrode is placed at the same level as the V_4 and V_5 electrodes, but in the mid axillary line which is an imaginary vertical line drawn from the middle of the armpit. Electrodes should be placed in regions with no or minimal hair as hair might prevent good contact between the skin and the electrode. Electrodes are not placed on bones because bony tissue does not conduct electrical activity as well as muscular issue. In women, the electrodes should generally be placed below the breast (closer to the heart) but if necessary can be placed on top of the breast if this position is closest to the standard electrode position. Misplacement of the chest electrodes will lead to significant changes in the ECG recordings.

Some experts have advocated additional chest leads that extend around the back of the torso (V_7–V_9) or to the right chest (V_4R, V_5R, and V_6R) to provide a more complete measurement of cardiac electrical activity. Although these additional lead positions may be extremely useful in certain specific situations, for the purposes of this discussion the reader should simply be aware that these additional electrode positions have been described and might be encountered in the hospital.

Often continuous ECG recordings are obtained while the patient is in the hospital to allow for rapid identification of cardiac problems. In this case, the 10 electrodes required for the standard ECG (4 on the limbs and 6 on the anterior chest) can be cumbersome for a patient to have on at all times so that depending on the system, 3 to 6 electrodes are placed on the torso. Specialized algorithms are then used to "derive" a full 12 lead ECG in some systems. Although these recording systems are useful for rapid evaluation of abnormal rhythms or marked changes on the ECG, the full 12 lead ECG using 10 separate electrodes is generally required for final interpretation of many abnormalities. For example, if a person in the hospital develops chest pain or a sustained abnormal heart rhythm, if possible, a standard 12 lead ECG should be obtained even if their cardiac rhythm is being monitored.

Electrodes and leads

In order to measure any kind of electrical activity, two electrodes are required so that the measuring device can measure the voltage difference between the two locations. The ECG has traditionally used 12 electrode pairs or leads to measure the cardiac activity of the heart.

The ECG leads are generally divided into the frontal leads that use the extremity electrodes and measure electrical activity in a vertical plane, and the precordial leads that use the six chest electrodes and measure electrical activity in a roughly horizontal plane. Historically, the first leads that were used are referred to by Roman numerals I, II, and III (Figure 1.2): Lead I measures the voltage difference between the left arm and the right arm electrodes (with the right arm the "negative" electrode), lead II measures the difference between the right arm and the left leg electrodes (with the right arm as the "negative" electrode), and lead III measures the difference between the left leg and the left arm (with the left arm as the "negative" electrode). The right leg electrode is used as a ground. The ground is important for defining the zero voltage since ECG leads measure voltage differences rather than absolute values. From a practical

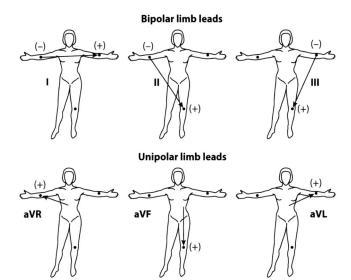

Figure 1.2:

The electrodes used for obtaining the frontal leads of the ECG: I, II, III, aVR, aVL, and aVF. Leads aVR, aVL, and aVF are often called the unipolar limb leads because they record the voltage change in one of the extremities relative to an averaged value of the other electrodes. (Reproduced with permission from FM Kusumoto, *Cardiovascular Pathophysiology*, Hayes Barton Press, Raleigh, NC, 2004.)

standpoint, the ECG machine uses the signal from the ground to help filter extraneous electrical noise. The other three frontal leads are referred to by the shorthand aVR, aVL, and aVF and one electrode (the positive electrode) at the right arm, left arm, and left leg respectively compared to a composite electrode that is the averaged voltage from the remaining two electrodes. The small letter "a" is for "augmented" since the signal obtained is augmented or larger because the second electrode used is an averaged voltage from the other two limb leads.

Since leads I, II, III, aVR, aVL, and aVF measure activity in the same plane they are always considered together and traditionally represented by a large circle with the negative electrodes for each of the leads aligned in the middle of the chest (Figure 1.3). The positive electrodes extend outward in

(a) **Frontal plane leads**

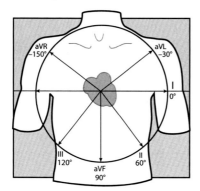

Frontal plane formed by leads I, II, and III and the three unipolar leads

(b) **Horizontal plane leads**

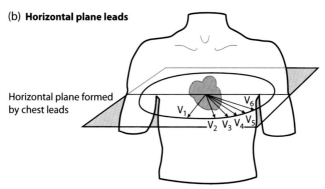

Horizontal plane formed by chest leads

Figure 1.3:

(a): the limb leads with the negative terminals aligned in the center of the torso fan out in a single plane called the frontal plane.

(b): The precordial leads with the negative terminal aligned in the center fan out in a horizontal plane that is perpendicular to the frontal plane. (Reproduced with permission from FM Kusumoto, *Cardiovascular Pathophysiology*, Hayes Barton Press, Raleigh, NC, 2004).

a circle in a single plane called the frontal plane. Specific orientations in the frontal plane are defined by the degrees of a circle with the horizontal axis toward the left is defined as 0° with positive values in the clockwise direction and negative values in the counterclockwise direction. In this way each of the extremity leads can be defined by a specific orientation: I, II, and III are 0°, 60°, and 120° respectively and aVR, aVL, and aVF are −150°, −30°, and 90° respectively. One way that can help you visualize this is a compass with North, East, South, and West equal to −90°, 0°, 90°, and 180°.

For the precordial leads electrical activity is measured between one of the six chest electrodes and the sum of the left arm, right arm, and left leg signals which is generally close to zero since the signals tend to cancel out (Figure 1.2). The composite electrode is considered the negative electrode and the electrode on the anterior chest as the positive electrode. With the negative electrode placed in the middle of the torso, the positive electrodes of the precordial leads fan out in a horizontal plane that is roughly perpendicular to the frontal plane (Figure 1.3).

Although truthfully voltage differences are measured between two electrodes, by convention the positive electrode of any electrode pair is used to indicate the general orientation of a specific lead. Don't get too wrapped up into positive and negative electrodes (as it does not help the clinician very much), it is easier to think of the positive electrode as the location of the "sensor" for a particular lead receiving input from the heart. Thinking in this fashion the 12 leads of the ECG in the frontal and horizontal planes provide a relatively comprehensive 3 dimensional "sensor net" for evaluating the electrical activity of the heart. One useful analogy is to compare the positive electrodes of an ECG to windows located on different walls of a building. By looking through all of the windows at the same time, the viewer ("peeping Tom?!") can get a fairly good idea of what is going on inside.

Clinically, the 12 leads can be grouped or divided based on the general orientation of the positive electrode relative to the heart (Figure 1.4). Leads II, III, and aVF are collectively called the "inferior leads" since they are oriented with the positive electrode "pointing upwards" and are in the best position measure electrical changes occurring on the bottom of the heart. Leads I, aVL, V_5, and V_6 are called the "lateral leads" since they best measure electrical activity on the left side of the heart, and leads V_1, V_2, V_3, and V_4 are called the "anterior leads." Sometimes leads V_1 and V_2 are further subclassified as "anteroseptal." Lead aVR is the only lead that is oriented on the right and best measures activity from the right side

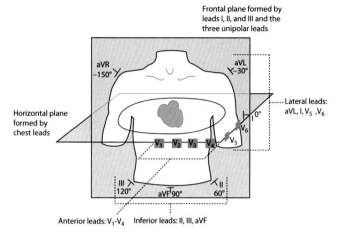

Frontal plane formed by
leads I, II, and III and the
three unipolar leads

aVR
−150°

aVL
−30°

Lateral leads:
aVL, I, V₅, V₆

Horizontal plane
formed by
chest leads

0°

V₆

V₁ V₂ V₃ V₄

V₅

III
120°

II
60°

aVF 90°

Anterior leads: V₁-V₄   Inferior leads: II, III, aVF

Figure 1.4:

Combining Figure 1.3A and 1.3B and showing the positive electrodes as "sensors." Notice that certain leads can be grouped together based on their general orientation relative to the heart: anterior, inferior, and lateral. (Adapted with permission from FM Kusumoto, *Cardiovascular Pathophysiology*, Hayes Barton Press, Raleigh, NC, 2004.)

(perhaps with a little contribution from leads III and V_1). Grouping the leads in this way is very helpful for identifying myocardial (heart muscle) injury and localizing the region of damage.

Since the positive electrodes of the leads are oriented in different positions around the heart, the shape of the deflections recorded on a lead will give the clinician some clue of the direction of depolarization. The electrical activity of cardiac cells is generally divided into two periods. When the cell is excited it is depolarized and this leads to contraction in heart cells. After a short period of time (about 0.4 seconds) the cell repolarizes and the heart cell relaxes. The terms depolarization and repolarization can sometimes be confusing but they come from the fact that at rest cells have a negative charge and when the cell is excited the charge is approximately zero (the cell has lost charge or has been *de*polarized).

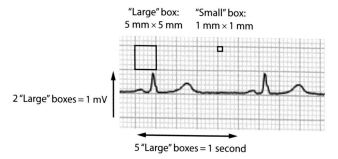

Figure 1.5:

ECG paper is divided into 1 mm × 1 mm "small" boxes that are grouped together in 5×5 mm "large" boxes. At standard settings, in the horizontal direction, 5 large boxes (25 mm) is equal to one second and, in the vertical direction 2 large boxes (10 mm) is equal to 1 mV.

Progressive activation of the heart cells leads to a wave of depolarization that is measured by the ECG. By convention, when depolarization travels toward the positive electrode a positive deflection is recorded and if the wave of depolarization is travelling away from the positive electrode a negative deflection will be recorded. Conversely if the direction of repolarization is oriented toward the positive electrode of an ECG lead a negative deflection will be recorded. To continue our earlier "window and building" analogy, we can think of the electrical activity of the heart as a person walking inside the building. As the person walks toward a window in the front of the building, he appears larger (and the electrical signal is positive), but from a window in the back, he is walking away so he looks smaller (and the electrical signal is negative). In the next chapter we will discuss the specific shapes of waves due to atrial and ventricular depolarization and ventricular repolarization (we will also explain why we cannot evaluate atrial repolarization).

Displaying the ECG

ECG recording paper is divided into "small boxes" that are 1mm by 1mm and "large boxes" that are 5mm by 5mm (Figure 1.5). Usually the ECG machine is set so that a 1 mV signal will lead to a 10mm deflection in the

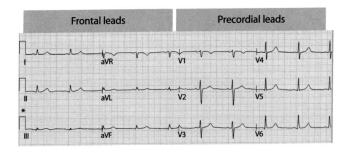

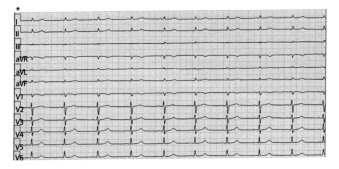

Figure 1.6:

Top: The most common standard display of the ECG shows the 12 leads as four columns and three rows. The first column displays leads I, II, and III. The second column displays aVR, aVL, and aVF. The third column displays V_1, V_2, and V_3. The fourth column displays V_4, V_5, and V_6. In this way the frontal leads are grouped as the first two columns and the precordial leads are grouped as the second two columns. A standardization mark (*) is always shown on the far left.

Bottom: A second standard display shows all of the leads one on top of another usually in the following order: I, II, III, aVR, aVL, aVF, V_1, V_2, V_3, V_4, V_5, and V_6. Both the top and the bottom ECGs are from the same person. Notice that the bottom ECG has smaller signals because it was recorded at "half standard." (Look at the standardization mark (*), a 1 mV signal made only a 5 mm signal.)

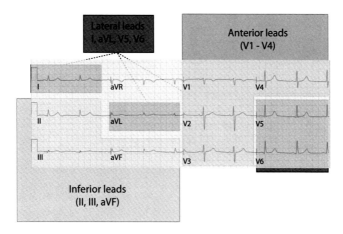

Figure 1.7:

Using the standard format combining Figure 1.4 and 1.6 that emphasizes and groups the ECG leads that look at similar areas of the heart: The inferior leads, the anterior leads, and the lateral leads.

ECG in the vertical direction. In the horizontal direction, the usual paper speed is 25 mm per second so that each large box (5 mm) represents 0.20 seconds and each little box (1 mm) represents 0.04 seconds. The settings of an ECG machine can generally be determined by looking for a standard mark usually at the far left of an ECG, where a 1 mV signal for 0.2 seconds is delivered. If the ECG machine is set to its usual settings this leads to a standardization mark signal that is 10 mm tall and 5 mm wide (Figure 1.6). If the paper speed is decreased to 12.5 mm per second, the signals become more compressed on the horizontal axis because each large box represents 0.40 seconds and if the paper speed is increased to 50 mm per second (10 large boxes equals one second), each large box is 0.10 seconds. In the same way if the voltage standard is halved then a 1 mV deflection leads to a 0.5 mm deflection and the size of the signal will be "squished" (Figure 1.6). In general these other settings are not used for the 12 lead ECG.

Although monitors still use specially designed paper that produces long "strips" of signals, for the sake of convenience and easier evaluation of all 12 leads, 12 lead ECGs are generally printed on standard letter size paper. Most commonly, the 12 lead ECG is displayed in four columns and three rows (Figure 1.6). The first column shows I, II, and III, the second column shows aVR, aVL, and aVF, the third column shows V_1, V_2, and V_3, and the fourth column shows V_4, V_5, and V_6. Just remember that the first two columns are frontal leads and the second two columns show the precordial leads. If the ECG is set at the standard paper speed, on standard letter paper, the full ECG records 10 seconds of electrical activity and each lead has 2.5 seconds of recording. A standard piece of paper is 279 mm long or about 55 "large" boxes. Another format usually called a rhythm strip shows a single lead for 10 seconds. Three to twelve leads are shown one on top of another (Figure 1.6).

Using the standard format, the inferior leads (II, III, and aVF) take up the "bottom left corner" of the ECG, the anterior leads (V1–V4) are in the "upper right corner", and the lateral leads (V5,V6, I, and aVL) are scattered all over (Figure 1.7).

CHAPTER 2

The Normal ECG

Before we can discuss the normal ECG, a quick review of the anatomy and the function of the heart is essential to provide a framework for our discussion. Unoxygenated blood from the body returns to the heart via the large superior and inferior *vena cavae*. Blood from these large veins enters into the right atrium and if the tricuspid valve is open the right atrium is a large passive "passage way." Atrial contraction causes a final surge of blood to fill the right ventricle and as the ventricles contract the tricuspid valve closes and the pulmonic valve opens and blood is expelled from the heart and is pumped to the lungs (Figure 2.1). Once oxygenated by the lungs the blood returns to the heart via the left atrium, and in a process similar to the right, blood flows fills the left ventricle both passively and actively when the left atrium contracts. When the left ventricle contracts, the mitral valve closes and the aortic valve opens and blood is expelled from the heart to the body. This process seems extremely complex but is actually fairly simple if we think about cardiac activity from two different vantage points. From the perspective of a single blood cell, blood travels sequentially through the *vena cavae*, right atrium, right ventricle, and pulmonary arteries to the lungs. Once oxygenated the blood cell travels through the pulmonary veins back to the left atrium, left ventricle, and finally is propelled into the aorta. From the perspective of heart cells, there is near simultaneous activation of the right and left atria and after a slight delay almost simultaneous activation of the right and left ventricles. This sequential pumping process is controlled by electrical signals generated by the heart that can be measured by the ECG.

ECG Interpretation for Everyone: An On-The-Spot Guide, First Edition.
Fred Kusumoto and Pam Bernath.
© 2012 John Wiley & Sons, Ltd. Published 2012 by John Wiley & Sons, Ltd.

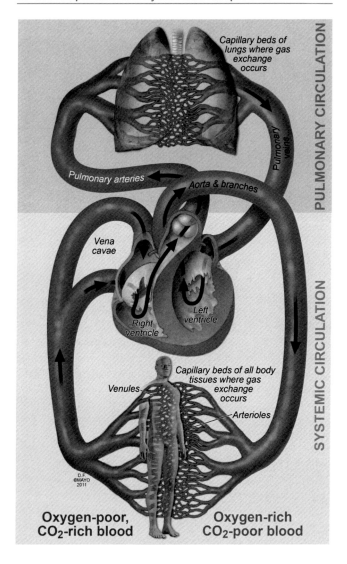

Capillary beds of lungs where gas exchange occurs

PULMONARY CIRCULATION

Pulmonary veins

Pulmonary arteries

Aorta & branches

Vena cavae

Left ventricle

Right ventricle

SYSTEMIC CIRCULATION

Capillary beds of all body tissues where gas exchange occurs

Venules

Arterioles

D.F.
©MAYO
2011

Oxygen-poor, CO₂-rich blood

Oxygen-rich CO₂-poor blood

Normal electrical activity of the heart
Atrial depolarization

Certain specialized cells exhibit spontaneous depolarization and are called "pacemaker" cells. Although cells in the AV node, His Purkinje system, and sometimes atrial and ventricular tissue exhibit spontaneous activity, since the rate of spontaneous depolarization is highest in a region called the sinus node, the sinus node generally serves as the principal pacemaker of the heart.

The sinus node is a small spindle shaped structure located at the junction of the superior *vena cava* and the right atrium. The sinus node has spontaneous pacemaker activity between 60–100 beats per minute. The sinus node receives nerve input from both the sympathetic and parasympathetic autonomic system and this is why the heart rate varies. With exercise, increased sympathetic input leads to an increase in the rate of spontaneous pacemaker activity that in turn will lead to faster depolarization of the atria and ventricles (and faster heart rates when you measure the peripheral pulse). At night, increased parasympathetic input leads to a slowing of the pacemaker rate. Sometimes this dynamic interplay can be observed during breathing. As a general rule, with slow inspiration the heart rate slows (check your own pulse) and with expiration the heart rate increases (particularly if you do not immediately take another breath). Although it initiates electrical activation, the sinus node is so small that the current it generates cannot be seen on the surface ECG (Figure 2.2).

Figure 2.1:

Basic diagram of blood circulation in the body. Deoxygenated blood returns to the heart from the body via the inferior and superior *vena cavae*. Blood enters the right atrium and sequential right atrial and right ventricular contraction pumps blood to the lungs via the pulmonary arteries. Blood is oxygenated in the lung and returns to the left atrium via the pulmonary veins. Sequential contraction of the left atrium and left ventricle pumps the oxygenated blood into the aorta. Blood is then distributed to the body and the cycle repeats. (Illustration by David Factor.)

(a)

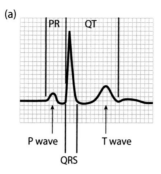

PR   QT

P wave   T wave

QRS

(b)

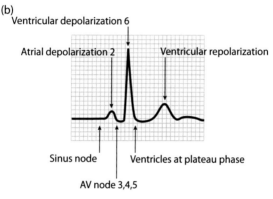

Ventricular depolarization 6

Atrial depolarization 2   Ventricular repolarization

Sinus node   Ventricles at plateau phase

AV node 3,4,5

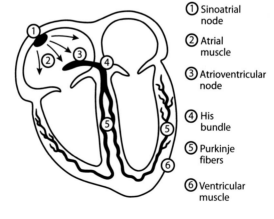

① Sinoatrial node

② Atrial muscle

③ Atrioventricular node

④ His bundle

⑤ Purkinje fibers

⑥ Ventricular muscle

The pacemaker activity produced by the sinus node is propagated through the atria, and since the sinus node is located "high and to the right," the right atrium is activated before the left atrium and the general direction of atrial depolarization is "high to low" and "right to left." Depolarization of the atrial tissue leads to release of Ca^{2+} ions from the *sarcoplasmic recticulum* in the cells of the atrium that in turn causes the heart cells to contract. On a larger scale, contraction of all of the atrial cells leads to contraction of the atrial chamber and provides the final filling of the right ventricle. It should be apparent that this is a fairly complex process and that there is a small but measurable delay between atrial depolarization and actual movement of blood (1. atrial cell is excited; 2. Ca^{2+} ions are released; 3. atrial cells (chambers) contract; and 4. blood moves). Electrical activity generated by atrial depolarization produces the P wave on the ECG.

Although depolarization of the sinus node cannot be seen on the ECG, evidence that the sinus node is generating the electrical impulse can be obtained by inspecting the shape of the P wave. If the sinus node is "driving" the heart, the P wave is negative in aVR and positive in lead II ("high to low" and "right to left"). Generally right atrial and left atrial depolarization proceed in the same direction so that in a given lead the P wave is positive or negative. Relook at Figure 1.6 from Chapter 1, and notice that the small P wave is generally either all negative (lead aVR) or predominantly positive (the rest of the leads). The common exception is lead V_1 (Figure 2.3). In this case, right atrial depolarization travels "toward" V_1 leading to an initial positive deflection, but sometimes a later negative deflection can be observed because of left atrial depolarization. In fact if you refer to Chapter 8, Figure 8.14 on left ventricular hypertrophy, you will see that a large negative deflection in lead V_1 is an important indicator of left atrial enlargement.

Right and left atrial depolarization is usually complete within 0.10 seconds so the normal P wave is 2–3 little boxes wide. The atria have a

Figure 2.2:

(a). The ECG deflections of the different portions of the heart and commonly measured intervals.

(b). The specific points where different portions of the heart are depolarized in relation to the surface ECG.

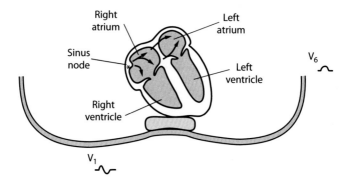

Figure 2.3:
Atrial depolarization relative to leads V_1 and V_6. Notice that since the sinus node is located in the right atrium, the right atrium is depolarized before the left atrium.

very small mass compared to the ventricles so the normal P wave is usually less than 2.5mm (two and a half little boxes) tall. Atrial repolarization generates voltages so small it is not seen on the ECG.

Atrioventricular conduction

(AV node, His bundle, bundle branches, and Purkinje system)

Once the atria are depolarized and the atria contract, blood is pumped into the right and left ventricles. As has been mentioned, the speed of electrical activity is much faster than the speed of blood, so to better improve the timing of atrial and ventricular *contraction*, the electrical impulse of atrial depolarization encounters the AV node where the con-duction velocity is slowed. At this point, the atria are completely depolar-ized and the ventricles are about to be depolarized. Since there is no electrical activity that can be measured by the ECG (the electrical impulse traveling through the very small AV node cannot be measured from the body surface), an isoelectric period can be observed on the ECG (Figure 2.2). The duration of the isoelectric period will depend at least in part on the speed of the electrical impulse through the AV node. For example, if the electrical impulse is abnormally slow through the AV node, a long isoelectric period will be observed.

After slow depolarization of the AV node, the velocity of activation speeds up as the impulse travels through the His Purkinje system. The

His Purkinje has several components (His bundle, right and left bundles, Purkinje tissue) but all have similar electrical properties and are able to rapidly conduct electrical impulses. The electrical impulse first travels through the common bundle or bundle of His (named for its discoverer Wilhelm His) and divides into a large left bundle that activates the left ventricle and a thinner right bundle that activates the right ventricle. The left bundle further divides into two major components: the left anterior fascicle and the left posterior fascicle. The terminal portions of these branching bundles and fascicles are a network of Purkinje tissues that spread out as a net in the interior surface of both the right and left ventricles. Although the His Purkinje system allows rapid conduction and is extensive, its overall mass is relatively small so activation of these tissues cannot be observed on the surface ECG. In fact, abnormalities of components of these systems are deduced because different portions of the ventricle are activated abnormally. In general, the normal His Purkinje system allows the electrical impulse to be "delivered" to large portions of the ventricle at nearly the same time so that right and left ventricular depolarization can start simultaneously and blood can be efficiently and forcefully expelled from the heart. If the His Purkinje system were not present or functioned abnormally some regions would contract before others and blood would not be pumped as efficiently.

Ventricular depolarization

Ventricular depolarization leads to a large deflection called the QRS complex. Ventricular depolarization has historically been called the QRS because it is made up of multiple components that are called Q waves, R waves, and S waves. Since describing the shape and the components of ventricular depolarization is very important, a common "language" for describing the QRS complex has been developed and is important to learn. Although the nomenclature can seem daunting, arbitrary, and confusing at first, it is actually easily learned and applied. The first negative deflection is called a Q wave, the first positive deflection an R wave, and any negative deflection after the R wave is called an S wave. Capital letters are used for large deflections and lower case letters for smaller deflections. In general larger deflections are produced because of larger mass or a more uniform direction of depolarization. If the ventricles are depolarized in several directions, the sum of their voltage as measured by the ECG will be smaller due to canceling out of activity. The decision on

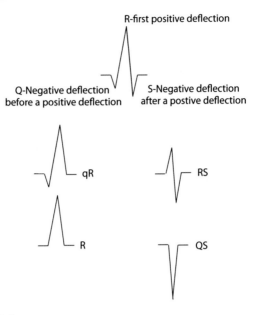

Figure 2.4:

Nomenclature for ventricular depolarization (QRS complex) and some examples. (Reproduced with permission from FM Kusumoto, ECG Interpretation: From Pathophysiology to Clinical Application, Springer, New York, NY, 2009.)

whether to use a capital letter or a lower case letter is often made by the clinician. A completely positive deflection is called an R wave and a completely negative complex is called a QS complex. Additional positive and negative deflections are described using a prime symbol: r' or s' depending on whether an additional positive or negative deflection is observed. Figure 2.4 shows some common complexes and their descriptors.

Normally the left ventricle has a larger mass than the right ventricle, so that even though the right and left ventricles are activated simultaneously the shape of the QRS complex is dominated by the left ventricle. For this reason, the general direction of ventricular depolarization in the frontal plane recorded by the limb leads is right to left and "high to low" (Figure 2.5).

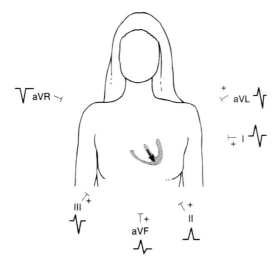

Figure 2.5:

The general direction of cardiac activation in the frontal plane is called the cardiac axis. The largest positive deflection will be recorded in the lead that is oriented most directly in the path of ventricular depolarization (in this case, lead II). (Adapted with permission from FM Kusumoto, *Cardiovascular Pathophysiology*, Hayes Barton Press, Raleigh, NC, 2004.)

The cardiac axis is used to more precisely calculate the direction of ventricular depolarization. The value of the axis is given in degrees using the lead alignment shown in Figures 1.3 and 1.4 in Chapter 1. A normal cardiac axis can have a wide range between −35° and 110° but is usually about 60°. The easiest way to calculate the cardiac axis is to remember that the ECG lead that is "looking" most directly at the wave of depolarization will have the largest positive deflection with smaller positive deflections recorded as the recording lead "looks" at the wave of depolarization from larger and larger angles. When the lead is perpendicular to the wave of depolarization a biphasic signal that is first positive and then negative is recorded (Figure 2.6). For most people, the

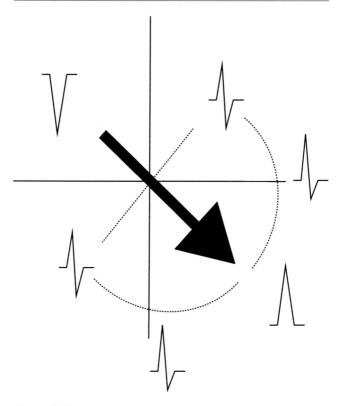

Figure 2.6:

The shape of the QRS complex will depend on the relationship between the wave of cardiac depolarization and the orientation of the lead. If the lead is directly in front of the depolarization wave a large positive signal will be recorded. As leads are oriented away from the wave of depolarization, the size of the positive wave will decrease and a terminal negative wave will be recorded as the wave of depolarization is traveling away from the lead. When a lead is perpendicular to the depolarization wave an equally biphasic wave will be recorded. When the wave of depolarization is directed away from the lead a negative deflection will be recorded.

largest QRS complex is observed in lead II and a completely negative QRS complex is often recorded in aVR (Figure 1.6 in Chapter 1).

If the axis is abnormally shifted to the right > 110° the largest positive wave will be recorded in lead III and if the axis is shifted to the left the largest R wave will be in aVL. Traditionally large sections of texts have been devoted to calculating the exact value of the QRS axis. Although useful for making sure someone knows the basis of ECGs, from a clinical standpoint estimating the general direction of ventricular depolarization is all that is required. The general direction of ventricular depolarization can be calculated by at least three different methods:

Find the lead with the largest QRS, and the mean electrical activation travels in the direction of the lead. If 2 leads are about the same height, the axis will be between these 2 leads.

Find the most isoelectric lead (most biphasic) and the largest QRS should be perpendicular to this lead. The lead with the largest QRS represents the general direction of the axis. Each limb lead has a corresponding perpendicular limb lead to form a pair: lead I and lead aVF; lead II and lead aVL; lead III and lead aVR.

The mean QRS axis can be calculated by the limb leads I and aVF. Keep in mind the four quadrants that are divided by 90 degrees.

- If lead I is positive and lead aVF is positive, the axis is normal because it falls between −30 to +110, which is the normal axis (normal quadrant).
- If lead I is positive, lead aVF is negative, and lead II is also negative, it falls between −30 and −90 which is left axis deviation (left quadrant).
- If lead I is negative and lead aVF is positive, this is a right axis deviation (right quadrant).
- If lead I is negative and lead aVF is negative, then this is extreme right axis deviation (northwest quadrant (using our compass analogy in the last chapter) or "no man's land").

Of these three methods, simply looking for the limb lead with the largest R wave is generally sufficient and the easiest method to remember. Although the QRS axis can be abnormal due to abnormalities of the heart, it is also important to remember that the cardiac axis reflects the

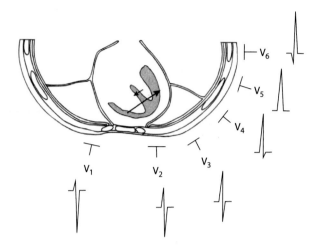

Figure 2.7:

In the horizontal plane, the precordial leads generally record two components of ventricular depolarization. First septal activation proceeds from left to tight and then a larger right to left wave of depolarization is observed since the left ventricle has much more mass than the right ventricle. This second component of ventricular activation is usually much larger than septal activation simply on the basis of mass (mass of the septum is small relative to the rest of the left ventricle).

position of the heart relative to the body so will also be affected by conditions that change the position of the heart within the thorax. For example, in chronic obstructive lung disease the heart may hang more vertically in the chest and this leads to a more rightward axis even in the absence of any abnormalities of the heart itself.

The shape of the QRS complex in the precordial leads can also vary with the relative orientation of the ventricles in the chest cavity. Generally the QRS complex in lead V_1 has an rS morphology. Initial septal activation occurs from left to right (because the left bundle branches off "first" compared to the right bundle) and since the left ventricle is usually positioned behind the right ventricle a large negative deflection is observed (Figure 2.7). In lead V_6, the QRS complex will often have a small q wave due to "left–to–right" septal activation followed by a large R wave due to left ventricular activation. Often the term R wave progression is used to describe the relative sizes of the R waves in the precordial leads. In lead V_1 and lead V_2 small r waves are present because they represent septal activation, but the R wave becomes larger laterally as it now represents left ventricular depolarization. The precordial leads where the R wave and S wave are approximately equal is called the transitional zone and usually occurs between leads V_2 and V_4, with lead V_3 being the most common site.

As has been mentioned, the His Purkinje system is important for allowing simultaneous left ventricular and right ventricular activation. This phenomenon can be seen in the ECG, despite the ventricle being significantly larger than the atria and thus the QRS has a larger amplitude than the P wave, the duration of the P wave and the QRS complex are normally fairly similar – generally a little less than three little boxes or ≤ 0.12 seconds.

ST segment

Once depolarized, the ventricles continue to contract for about 0.4 to 0.45 seconds to allow blood to be expelled from the heart to the lungs or body. During this period, the ventricular cells are in their plateau phase (they remain depolarized) so there are usually no electrical gradients that can be measured by the ECG so that after the QRS complex there is an isoelectric period often called the ST segment. As we will see later, changes in the ST segment are important for identifying myocardial injury and ischemia.

Ventricular repolarization

As ventricular contraction is completed, the ventricles begin to repolarize and return to their baseline state to prepare for another depolarization/contraction sequence. Ventricular repolarization produces the T wave. Ventricular repolarization is much more heterogeneous when compared to ventricular depolarization (which is mediated by the His Purkinje system) and this leads to a T wave that is more broad based and generally of lower amplitude (think "squashed") when compared to the QRS complex. It is an interesting paradox that the normal T wave generally is in "the same direction" as the direction of the QRS complex because depolarization proceeds from endocardium to epicardium ("inside–out") and repolarization proceeds in the opposite direction from epicardium to endocardium ("outside–in") (Figure 2.8). Part of the basis for this apparent

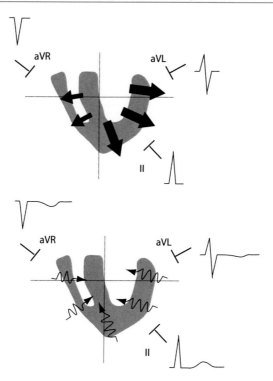

Figure 2.8:

Depolarization (*Top*) and repolarization (*Bottom*) of the ventricles as observed in the frontal plane. Depolarization occurs almost simultaneously because of the His Purkinje system. Depolarization occurs from endocardium to epicardium and since the left ventricle has a larger mass than the right ventricle the overall direction of depolarization is from right to left and from the superior portion of the ventricles to the lower portion of the ventricles. In general this leads to an axis of approximately 60° so that a large R wave is noted in lead II, an RS complex is observed in aVL (depolarization travels toward and then away from this lead), and a QS complex is noted in lead aVR. Depolarization occurs from epicardium to endocardium in a more gradual fashion. This leads paradox is that the epicardial cells have a shorter action potential duration than endocardial cells.

Timing of normal cardiac activity

In the first section of this chapter we focused on the shape of the various waveforms but one of the important uses for the ECG is measuring the timing relationship of different cardiac events.

Heart rate (R–R interval)

The most basic timing measurement of the ECG is the heart rate. Since the pulse is generated by ventricular contraction, the distance between two QRS complexes (the R–R interval) will provide an estimate of the heart rate. Remember that each large box represents 0.20 seconds so slower heart rates will be associated with larger distances between QRS complexes. For example if the heart rate is 60 beats per minute, QRS complexes will occur once every second and the QRS complexes will be separated by 5 large boxes at the standard paper speed. If the heart rate is 100 beats per minute only 3 large boxes or 0.60 seconds will separate each QRS complex. One can do the math and calculate the exact heart rate by using the formula:

Heart rate (beats per minute) = 60 / (the R–R interval in seconds)

This formula is accurate but can be rather cumbersome (and hard to remember) in clinical medicine. Since the importance of determining the exact heart rate is rarely clinically important, it is much easier to estimate the rate by the following formula (Figure 2.9):

Heart rate (beats per minute) = 300 / (the number of large boxes between two QRS complexes)

Figure 2.8: (*Cont'd*)
to an upright T wave in II, a flat (slightly inverted in this example) in lead aVL, and an inverted T wave in aVR. Notice that since repolarization is generally in the opposite direction than depolarization, the QRS and T wave orientation is usually the same. (Reproduced with permission from FM Kusumoto, *ECG Interpretation: From Pathophysiology to Clinical Application*, Springer, New York, NY, 2009.)

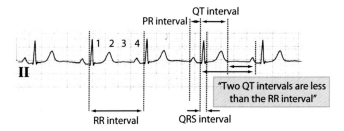

Figure 2.9:

Calculation of rate and common intervals. In this case the QRS complexes are separated by 4 large boxes (R–R interval) so the rate is approximately 75 bpm (300/4). The PR interval is measured from the beginning of the P wave to the beginning of the QRS complex. The QRS interval is measured from the beginning of the QRS complex to the end of the QRS complex. The QT interval is measured from the beginning of the QRS complex to the end of the T wave. In general the QT is normal if it less than half the R–R interval ("You can fit two QTs into one R–R"). (Reproduced with permission from FM Kusumoto, *ECG Interpretation: From Pathophysiology to Clinical Application*, Springer, New York, NY, 2009.)

So that if the QRS complexes are separated by two large boxes the heart rate is 150 bpm, three large boxes yields a heart rate of 100 bpm, four large boxes 75 bpm, and five large boxes 60 bpm. Finally, another very simple way to estimate the rate is to remember that at a standard paper speed of 25 mm/s most 12 lead ECGs record 10 seconds of cardiac activity. Simply count the number of beats and multiply by 6.

In most cases the rate of atrial activity will be the same as the rate calculated from ventricular depolarization (R–R interval) since the sinus node is normally the "driver" of the heart and the AV node/bundles conduct every atrial impulse to the ventricles. In some cases the atrial rate will be slower than the ventricular rate either due to more rapid ventricular depolarization or slower atrial activity due to abnormalities in sinus node function. In both of these conditions there will be more QRS

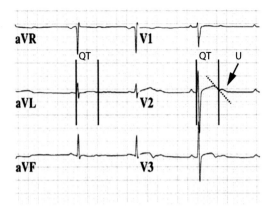

Figure 2.10:
Measurement of the QT interval. The end of the T wave is best calculated by drawing a tangent line along the steepest portion of the T wave. In this case a prominent U wave is observed that should not be included in the measurement of the QT interval.

complexes than P waves. Conversely, sometimes the atrial rate will be more rapid than the ventricular rate because atrioventricular conduction does not maintain a 1:1 relationship between atrial depolarization and ventricular depolarization (more P waves than QRS complexes).

PR interval
The PR interval is measured from the beginning of the P wave to the beginning of the QRS complex (Figure 2.2). The PR interval provides an estimate of atrioventricular conduction and represents right atrial depolarization (remember AV node conduction usually begins near the end of right atrial depolarization and at the same time left atrial depolarization begins since the AV node is located in the interatrial septum between the right and left atria), AV node depolarization, and His Purkinje depolarization. The normal PR interval gets longer with age, but for adults is ≤ 0.20 seconds and is most commonly about 0.16 s (4 little boxes).

QRS interval

The QRS interval is measured from the beginning of the QRS complex to the end of the QRS complex and provides a rough estimate of the time required for depolarization between the first portions of the ventricle to be activated to the last portion of the ventricle to be depolarized. The normal QRS interval is ≤ 0.12 seconds (3 little boxes). Generally, the posterior portion of the left ventricle closest to the spine is the last ventricular site to depolarize although this can change if there is blocked conduction in either the left or right bundle. In fact, the hallmark for identifying block in one of the bundles is a widened QRS interval > 0.12 seconds (Chapter 7, Figures 7.1 and 7.2; Chapter 8, Figures 8.1 and 8.2).

QT interval

The last commonly measured interval is the QT interval. The QT interval is measured from the beginning of the QRS complex to the end of the T wave. The end of the T wave can sometimes be difficult to measure because the T wave has a much more gradual upslope and downslope but drawing a tangent line along the steepest part of the descending portion of the T wave has been advocated and accepted as the best way to measure the QT interval (Figure 2.10). Most commonly the QT interval is measured in lead II although recent guidelines recommend using the lead with the longest QT interval (usually lead V_2 or V_3). Measurement of the QT interval in leads V_2 and V_3 can be sometimes be more difficult to measure because of a U wave. A U wave is a very low amplitude signal that is probably due to rapid filling of the ventricles rather than another wave of repolarization. It is usually seen as a positive wave in leads V_2 and V_3 and is more commonly seen with slower heart rates. Although there has been some disagreement in the past, since the U wave does not appear to be due to ventricular repolarization most now agree that it should not be included in the measurement of the QT interval. The QT interval measures the time between the first ventricular cell to depolarize and the last ventricular cell to repolarize, and provides a rough estimate of the duration of the plateau phase of ventricular tissue. As described in Chapter 6, Figures 6.7–6.14, the QT interval is prolonged in patients with electrolyte disorders, certain medications, and may be congenitally long due to abnormalities of K^+ channels. The QT interval is longer in women and decreases with rate. For this reason the QT interval is usually corrected to rate by an algorithm and called the

QTc where "c" stands for "corrected." The most common method for correcting the QT interval for rate is the Bazett's formula:

$QTc = QT \text{ (seconds)} / (R-R)^{1/2}$

Where "R–R" is the R–R interval in seconds. Several other techniques for rate correction have been suggested but the Bazett's correction is the most commonly used and the one provided by most automated ECG algorithms. A QTc > 450 s in men or > 460 s in women have been used as cut–off values for dividing normal and abnormal values but it should be remembered that in reality the QTc can vary from many causes and there is significant overlap in QTc intervals between patients with known genetic disorders that cause QTc prolongation and the normal population. An easy way to "get a feel" on whether the QT interval is prolonged is to remember that in general the QT interval should be less than half the R–R interval. Given the obvious difficulty in measuring the QT interval it is not surprising that even cardiologists, who are physicians that specialize in heart diseases, often incorrectly measure the QT interval.

CHAPTER 3

ECG Interpretation Basics

Now we come to the art of evaluating the ECG and using it in clinical context. Although computer analysis of the ECG has become far more accurate over the past two decades, the ability to carefully interpret an ECG remains an important skill in clinical medicine. However, although the ECG may be extremely useful, it is important to remember that, at best, the ECG provides supplementary information to a careful history and physical examination.

Traditionally ECG interpretation is taught by sequentially calculating the heart rate, measuring the cardiac axis, measuring cardiac intervals, evaluating the P wave, the QRS complex, the ST segment, and then the T wave. However, in clinical practice we appropriately focus on identifying potential life-threatening problems first. In fact, we believe that, in general, most of clinical training focuses on being able to distinguish "very, very" sick from "not-so" sick. In these emergent and urgent situations the ECG is really useful for 1) evaluating abnormally fast and slow heart rates and 2) identifying myocardial injury.

With this in mind, use the algorithm in Figure 3.1 for your initial analysis of the ECG. First, make an initial assessment of the heart rhythm. Make sure that P waves are present and that every P wave results in a QRS complex, and, most important, that the overall heart rate is between 50 and 110 beats per minute. If these statements are true, then the heart rhythm is not life-threatening (although not necessarily normal). The point here is that any heart rhythm with these characteristics (P waves and QRS complexes with a 1:1 relationship at a normal rate) should be able to provide sufficient blood flow to the lungs, brain, and the rest of the peripheral circulation. Second, the ST segment after the QRS complex should be evaluated. The ST segment should be isoelectric – in other words, the segment separating the T wave and

ECG Interpretation for Everyone: An On-The-Spot Guide, First Edition.
Fred Kusumoto and Pam Bernath.
© 2012 John Wiley & Sons, Ltd. Published 2012 by John Wiley & Sons, Ltd.

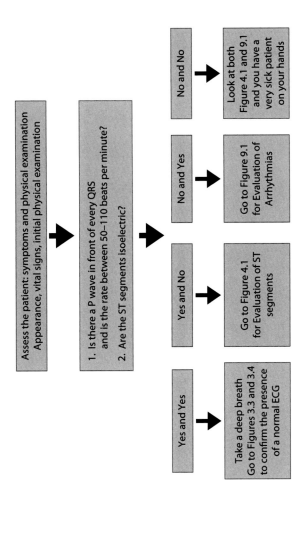

Figure 3.1:
Basic algorithm for rapid identification of serious arrhythmias or serious myocardial injury.

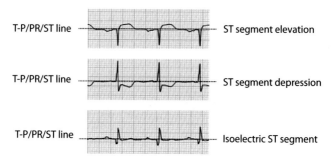

Figure 3.2:

Evaluation of the ST segment. Use the T–P and PR segment (dotted line) to estimate the level of an isoelectric ST segment. ST segment elevation is an ST segment above this imaginary line, ST segment depression is an ST segment below this line, and an isoelectric ST interval will be level and near this line.

the P wave of the next beat (sometimes called the T–P interval and the period when the ventricle is filling "passively" without atrial contraction), the PR interval, and the ST segment should all be at the same level (Figure 3.2). If the ST segment is elevated or depressed, particularly if the patient is also complaining of chest pain or shortness of breath, myocardial injury may be present. No mystery, no voodoo, and no hocus pocus: probably 90–95% of emergent conditions in which the ECG provides rapid information that requires immediate clinical treatment is addressed by evaluating these two issues. If the rhythm is normal and the ST segments are isoelectric ("Yes and Yes"), interpretation of the ECG can take a more leisurely pace once the patient has been attended to.

It is important to remember that a comprehensive analysis of the ECG can have many components (Figure 3.3). In general, although all of these components fall into three major groups: Evaluation of the rhythm (Chapters 9–11), evaluation of ventricular depolarization (Chapters 7 and 8), and evaluation of ventricular repolarization (Chapters 4–6). The characteristics of a normal ECG are illustrated in Figure 3.4.

Yes and Yes

Components of ECG interpretation	Normal findings
Rhythm identification (Chapter 9)	Upright P wave in II PR interval <0.20 s
Evaluate ventricular depolarization (Chapter 7)	QRS narrow and negative in V1 Normal cardiac axis (−30° to 110°) No abnormal Q waves Normal QRS voltage
Evaluate ventricular repolarization (Chapter 4)	"Normal" T waves Normal QT interval (QTc < 0.45s M , < 0.47s W)

Figure 3.3:

Once a life-threatening arrhythmia is ruled out and the presence of isoelectric ST segments is confirmed, the ECG can be evaluated in a systematic fashion. Although there are many components to a comprehensive interpretation of the ECG that are beyond the scope of this introductory text, in general there are three essential parts to ECG analysis. First, the rhythm should be specifically identified. We have already done some "triage" by identifying abnormally slow or fast heart rhythms. Second, ventricular depolarization should be assessed. ECG findings suggestive of abnormal ventricular depolarization include a wide QRS complex (> 0.12 s), a QRS complex that is positive in lead V_1, abnormal cardiac axis, and the presence of Q waves. Third, ventricular repolarization should be evaluated. Again, the reader has already done some triage by evaluating the ST segment but other abnormalities of ventricular repolarization include abnormal T waves (both inverted and peaked) and delayed ventricular repolarization (prolonged QT interval).

The normal ECG

1. Rate should be between 50 and 110 bpm

2. A P before every QRS (Positive P in lead II)

3. The QRS in V1 (MCL 1) should be narrow and negative (rS)

4. The ST segment should be isoelectric

5. The T wave should be the same direction as the QRS

Figure 3.4:

The characteristics of a normal ECG. First, the P wave is upright in lead II and negative in aVR suggesting that the atria are being depolarized by the sinus node. Every P wave is followed by a QRS complex with a PR interval of <.20 s, these two findings confirm that the AV node is functioning normally. Second, ventricular depolarization is characterized by a narrow QRS complex (<0.12 seconds), which suggests that the His Purkinje system is functioning normally with simultaneous activation of the right and left ventricles. The cardiac axis is approximately 60° with the largest positive deflection in the limb leads identified in lead II. The precordial QRS complexes are normal with a predominantly negative QRS complex in lead V_1. A Q wave in lead aVR (and sometimes in III) is expected since ventricular depolarization is traveling away from this lead and small Q waves (< 0.04 ms) due to septal activation can be seen in the lateral leads, particularly V_6. Repolarization is normal with an isoelectric ST segment and T waves that are in the same general direction as the QRS in that lead. The QT interval is normal and less than half the R–R interval.

CHAPTER 4

Abnormal Repolarization: ST Segment Elevation

You have come to this chapter in two ways. Either you identified ST segments that are not isoelectric or you have identified abnormal T waves (Figure 4.1). The ST segment and the T wave correlate with the plateau phase and repolarization of ventricular myocytes respectively and are particularly important for evaluation of the patient with chest pain or other symptoms suggestive of myocardial injury/ischemia (ischemia means that an organ is not receiving adequate amounts of blood and comes from the Greek word *iskhaimos*: *iskhein*: "To hold back" and *haima*: "blood"). It is important to remember that all three of these repolarization changes (ST segment elevation, ST segment depression, and T wave changes) can sometimes be observed on a single ECG and are often related. Clinically ST segment elevation requires the most urgent treatment and should always be the primary focus of the evaluation. In other words, the leads that display ST segment elevation directs you to the location and type of problem ("Where the money is"). If the ECG has ST segment elevation, use the figures in this chapter to help you with the diagnosis. If the ECG has ST depression only, recheck to make sure there are no leads with ST elevation and go to Chapter 5, and if the ST segments are isoelectric and only the T waves are inverted, go to Chapter 6. Very subtle ST segment elevation can be a normal finding in any lead, particularly in V_2 and V_3. However, any ST segment elevation > 2 mm in leads V_2 or V_3 or ST segment elevation > 1 mm in any of the other leads should be considered suspicious for a cardiac abnormality. Use Table 4.1 to decide whether: 1) The ST segment elevation is abnormal? and 2) Is the abnormal ST segment elevation due to myocardial injury?

ECG Interpretation for Everyone: An On-The-Spot Guide, First Edition.
Fred Kusumoto and Pam Bernath.
© 2012 John Wiley & Sons, Ltd. Published 2012 by John Wiley & Sons, Ltd.

ST segment Elevation (Figures 4.4–4.29)

Location

    Precordial leads (anterior, lateral or both)

    Inferior leads

    Both inferior and precordial leads

    Lead aVR

Reciprocal ST segment depression other than aVR

Accompanying Q waves

ST segment Depression (Figures 5.1–5.8)

T wave changes

    T wave inversion (Chapter 5)

    Prominent T waves (Chapter 5)

    Prolonged QT interval (Chapter 6)

Figure 4.1:

Evaluation of abnormal repolarization. If ST segment elevation is present the specific lead location(s) of the ST segment elevation should be identified. ST segment elevation associated with myocardial infarction is localized to one of the regions supplied by the major coronary arteries (see Figure 4.3). In addition to the localization of the ST segment elevation to a particular region supplied by a coronary artery, the presence of ST segment depression in other leads (so called reciprocal ST segment depression) or Q waves suggests myocardial injury as the cause of the ST segment elevation. Other repolarization abnormalities include ST segment depression (usually seen in the lateral leads), or abnormal T waves (See Chapters 5 and 6).

Table 4.1: Factors determining whether abnormal ST segment is present and whether abnormal ST segment elevation is more likely due to ischemia

---

Is abnormal ST segment elevation present?
(*Yes to any questions means abnormal*)
- Is ST segment elevation > 2 mm in V_2 and V_3, or > 1 mm in the other leads?
- Is the ST segment elevation present in two "adjacent" (contiguous) leads?

Is the abnormal ST segment elevation due to myocardial injury?
(*Yes to any questions means that myocardial injury is a likely cause*)
- Does the ST segment elevation correspond to a region supplied by a coronary artery (anterior, lateral, inferior)?
- Is reciprocal ST segment depression present?
- Are the T waves also inverted?
- Are Q waves present?

ST segment elevation is the hallmark ECG finding for patients who have total occlusion of one of the major coronary arteries that supply blood to the heart (Figure 4.2). In this case continued myocardial injury can lead to myocardial infarction (MI)-more commonly called a "heart attack." (The word infarction comes from the Latin word "*infarcire*" which means to "plug up.") The main reason for quickly identifying the presence of ST segment elevation is that several landmark studies have demonstrated the importance of reestablishing blood flow via either drugs to dissolve the clot (thrombolysis) or mechanically opening the artery (usually by taking the patient directly to the cardiac catheterization laboratory where cardiologists can restore blood flow with a variety of special techniques including balloons that dilate the narrowed area). In fact the data is so compelling for STEMI or "ST segment elevation myocardial infarction," hospitals in the United States are now being "graded" on the timeliness and their response to this condition. Myocardial infarction can also occur in the setting of ST segment depression and T wave changes (usually T wave inversion), and the clinical term for these conditions is NSTEMI or "non ST segment elevation myocardial infarction." The terms ischemia, injury, and infarction have traditionally been used to distinguish increasing degrees of severity based on ECG findings. "Ischemia" was characterized by ST segment depression

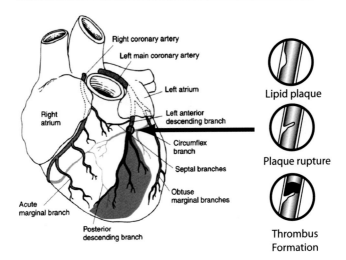

Lipid plaque

Plaque rupture

Thrombus
Formation

Figure 4.2:

Schematic for the development of myocardial ischemia/injury/infarction. A lipid plaque ruptures and thrombus (blood clot) forms at the exposed tissue/lipid. If the thrombus completely occludes flow, the patient develops a myocardial infarction (usually characterized by ST segment elevation) in the downstream myocardium (shaded area). Sometimes the clot does not completely occlude blood flow, but severe limitation of flow prevents sufficient blood to be supplied to the affected area (ischemia). (Adapted with permission from FM Kusumoto, *Cardiovascular Pathophysiology*, Hayes Barton Press, Raleigh, NC, 2004.)

or T wave changes, "Injury" was characterized by ST segment elevation without Q waves, and "Infarction" characterized by abnormal Q waves and ST segment elevation or depression. Now the diagnosis of myocardial damage is generally made by identifying abnormal amounts of cardiac proteins such as troponins in the blood. But the ECG is still used to distinguish myocardial infarctions associated with ST segment elevation (STEMI) and myocardial infarctions with any other ECG findings (NSTEMI).

One of the important hallmarks of ST segment elevation associated with a MI is localization of the ST segment elevation to a specific anatomic distribution. In most people there are three major coronary arteries that supply blood to the heart (Figure 4.3). The right coronary artery supplies blood to the inferior wall. The left main coronary artery almost immediately (usually within 1 or 2 cm) splits into a left anterior descending coronary artery supplies blood to the anterior wall, and a circumflex coronary artery supplies blood to the lateral wall. Complete occlusion of a coronary artery will generally lead to ST segment elevation in the leads that "look" directly at these areas. In many cases "reciprocal" ST depression will be observed in the other leads. The presence of a Q wave (initial negative deflection in the QRS complex) in a lead with ST segment elevation is very suggestive that a myocardial infarction is present.

As will be illustrated in the rest of the chapter, MI is associated with ST segment elevation in groups of leads (anterior: V_1 to V_4; inferior: II, III, and aVF; lateral: I, aVL, V_5 and V_6), depending on the site and extent of injury. As a corollary to this point, ST segment elevation due to myocardial infarction should be observed in several leads within a given lead group. Another commonly used way of emphasizing this important point is that significant ST segment elevation should be observed in two contiguous leads (leads that are roughly adjacent to each other). For further evaluation of ST segment elevation, it is easiest to consider the location (s) of the ST elevation: precordial (anterior and lateral), Inferior, both precordial and inferior, and only in aVR.

One specific point about anterior ST segment elevation requires special emphasis. Anterior ST segment elevation, particularly in leads V_1 through V_3, can be present in almost any condition that is associated with a wide negative QRS complex in lead V_1. The most common example is left bundle branch block. The specific ECG characteristics of conditions associated with a wide QRS complex are covered more extensively in Chapter 7, but in general anything that causes abnormal ventricular depolarization will cause abnormal repolarization including changes in the ST segment that can make evaluation of ST segments extremely problematic and often useless. As always the clinician should make decisions based on the patient's symptoms and "Hope for the best, but prepare for the worst."

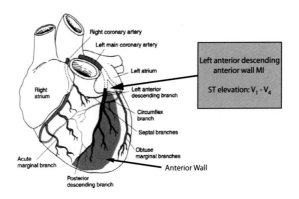

Right coronary artery

Left main coronary artery

Left atrium

Right atrium

Left anterior descending branch

Circumflex branch

Septal branches

Obtuse marginal branches

Acute marginal branch

Posterior descending branch

Anterior Wall

Left anterior descending anterior wall MI

ST elevation: $V_1 - V_4$

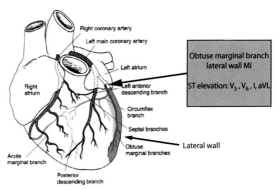

Right coronary artery

Left main coronary artery

Left atrium

Right atrium

Left anterior descending branch

Circumflex branch

Septal branches

Obtuse marginal branches

Acute marginal branch

Posterior descending branch

Lateral wall

Obtuse marginal branch lateral wall MI

ST elevation: V_5, V_6, I, aVL

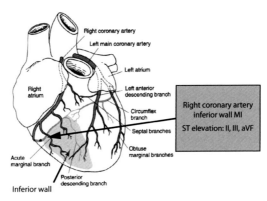

Right coronary artery

Left main coronary artery

Left atrium

Right atrium

Left anterior descending branch

Circumflex branch

Septal branches

Obtuse marginal branches

Acute marginal branch

Posterior descending branch

Inferior wall

Right coronary artery inferior wall MI

ST elevation: II, III, aVF

Figure 4.3:
Localization of ST segment elevation in relationship to the affected coronary artery that is occluded. If the left anterior descending artery is occluded ST segment elevation is usually seen in the anterior leads V_1–V_4. In most people the circumflex artery often has one or two large obtuse marginal arteries and occlusion of one of these arteries leads to a lateral wall myocardial infarction. ST segment elevation is usually seen in the lateral leads I, aVL, V_5, and V_6. The right coronary artery supplies the inferior wall in most people, so that occlusion leads to an inferior wall myocardial infarction. ST segment elevation is observed in the inferior leads II, III, and aVF.

Precordial ST Segment Elevation

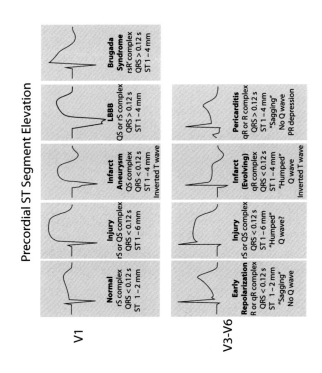

V1

Normal	Injury	Infarct Aneurysm	LBBB	Brugada Syndrome
rS complex	rS or QS complex	QS complex	QS or rS complex	rsR' complex
QRS < 0.12 s	QRS < 0.12 s	QRS < 0.12 s	QRS > 0.12 s	QRS > 0.12 s
ST 1–2 mm	ST 1–6 mm	ST 1–4 mm	ST 1–4 mm	ST 1–4 mm
		Inverted T wave		

V3–V6

Early Repolarization	Injury	Infarct (Evolving)	Pericarditis
R or qR complex	rS or QS complex	qR complex	qR or R complex
QRS < 0.12 s	QRS < 0.12 s	QRS < 0.12 s	QRS < 0.12 s
ST 1–2 mm	ST 1–6 mm	ST 1–4 mm	ST 1–4 mm
"Sagging"	"Humped"	"Humped"	"Sagging"
No Q wave	Q wave?	Q wave	No Q wave
		Inverted T wave	PR depression

Figure 4.4:

When precordial ST segment elevation is observed it is extremely useful to 1) look specifically at V_1 and 2) evaluate the specific precordial leads that have ST segment elevation. If the QRS in lead V_1 is wide and predominantly negative left bundle branch block may be present and accompanying ST segment elevation is very common. In fact ECG identification of myocardial infarction in the presence of left bundle branch block can be extremely problematic (Figure 4.27). A much rarer finding is the presence of Brugada Syndrome that is characterized by a terminal positive deflection (r' wave) and ST segment elevation in V_1 (Figures 4.15 and 4.16). In situations where the ST segment elevation is only present in the anterior leads (V_1 through V_4) the differential diagnosis is generally fairly limited. Isolated ST segment elevation in V_1 through V_3 can be seen as a normal variant, particularly in young men but is usually less than 2 mm. The ST segment elevation associated with an anterior wall myocardial infarction may be extremely prominent, sometimes > 5 mm and has often been described as having a "humped" shape and may obscure even large T waves. The presence of a Q wave (initial negative deflection or notch) in any of the anterior leads V_1–V_4 is abnormal and is evidence for a myocardial infarction. ST segment elevation in the lateral precordial leads V_5 and V_6 are associated with some additional possibilities. A specific pattern called early repolarization (Figure 4.6) is associated with lateral ST segment elevation and prominent T waves and is particularly common in African American men. In addition, pericarditis (Figure 4.21) a condition where there is acute inflammation of the sac surrounding the heart can also cause ST segment elevation.

Precordial ST Segment Elevation

"Normal" ST segment elevation
Not due to myocardial Injury

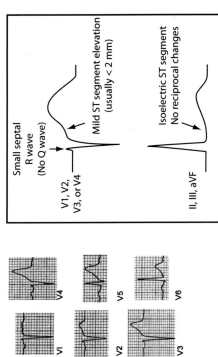

Small septal
R wave
(No Q wave)

Mild ST segment elevation
(usually < 2 mm)

V1, V2,
V3, or V4

Isoelectric ST segment
No reciprocal changes

II, III, aVF

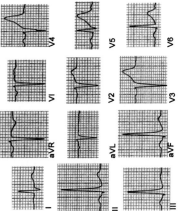

I

II

III

aVR

aVL

aVF

V1

V2

V3

V4

V5

V6

Figure 4.5:

Background: Precordial ST segment elevation may be observed, particularly in young men.

ECG: Anterior ST segment elevation < 2 mm in leads V_2 or V_3 (< 2.5 mm in men younger than 40 years old) may be a normal finding. "Normal" ST segment elevation will not be associated with abnormal Q waves and reciprocal ST segment depression will not be observed.

Clinical Issues: The presence of "normal" ST segment elevation does not change clinical prognosis.

Precordial ST Segment Elevation

"Normal" ST segment elevation due to early repolarization

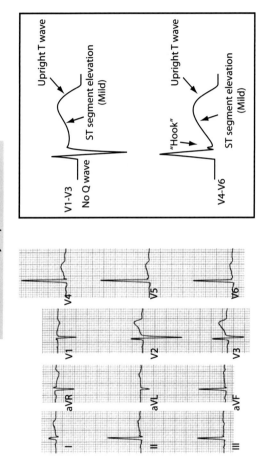

Figure 4.6:

Background: This is a normal variant in young men, particularly African Americans.

ECG: The ST changes are most prominent in the anterolateral leads. The J point (the junction between the QRS and the ST segment) will be elevated > 1 mm in at least 2 of the right precordial leads in 90% of young men. The ST segment will have a concave upward, slightly sagging appearance between the J point and the T wave, usually in the precordial leads V_2 to V_6. It is often greatest in V4. The ST segment elevation ranges from 0.5 mm to 5 mm, but it is usually <2 mm in the precordial leads and <0.5 mm in the limb leads. A notch (or hook) at the terminal portion of the QRS complex is frequently observed and Q waves are not present.

Clinical Issues: Early repolarization is usually benign, but there are some small studies that suggest that early repolarization may be slightly more common in patients with sudden cardiac death due to ventricular arrhythmias when compared to the general population. Currently there are no tests that can be used to identify the very small group of patients with early repolarization who may be at higher risk.

Precordial ST Segment Elevation Anterior Leads

Due to QRS widening from Bundel Branch Block
Not due to myocardial Injury

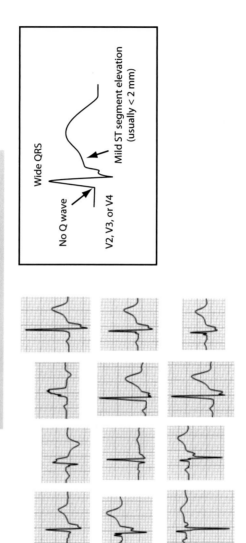

Wide QRS

Mild ST segment elevation
(usually < 2 mm)

No Q wave

V2, V3, or V4

Figure 4.7:

Background: Almost any condition that is associated with abnormal depolarization can be associated with minor ST segment changes.

ECG: In this example of a patient with abnormal conduction in his bundles (right bundle branch block and left anterior fascicular block) ST segment elevation is observed in V_2 and V_3. When abnormal depolarization due to bundle branch

block is present ST segment elevation may be observed in any lead where the QRS is entirely negative, or as in this case, where the terminal portion of the QRS is negative).

Clinical Issues: No specific treatment for the ST segment changes is required although the presence of bundle branch block can be associated with an increased risk of future problems with bradycardia.

Precordial ST Segment Elevation

Anterior Wall Myocardial Infarction

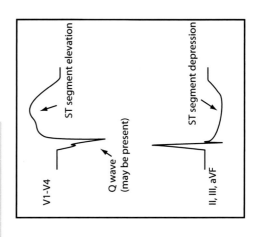

V1-V4

ST segment elevation

Q wave
(may be present)

ST segment depression

II, III, aVF

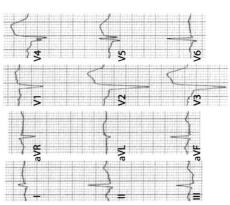

Figure 4.8:

Background: Occlusion of the left anterior descending coronary artery can cause a number of different patterns of ST segment elevation depending on the site of occlusion and the patient's individual anatomy. Although most people have three major arteries, the branching pattern of smaller arteries from these major branches can vary significantly from person to person.

ECG: An anterior wall myocardial infarction is associated with ST segment elevation in the precordial leads, usually most prominent in V_2 through V_4. There should be ST segment elevation in 2 adjacent anterior leads in order to make the diagnosis of Anterior MI. In this case ST segment elevation is also seen in V_5 and subtle ST segment elevation is also present in the lateral leads I and aVL. In general, for any type of myocardial infarction the extent of ST segment elevation provides a clue on the size of the myocardial

infarction: More leads with ST segment elevation = Larger myocardial infarction. The presence of a Q wave in the anterior leads is abnormal and is very strong evidence for a myocardial infarction. In some cases, particularly early in the course of a myocardial infarction Q waves will not be observed. In this example abnormal Q waves in V_1 to V_5 and aVL are present. A slender Q wave is noted in V_6 but since it is less than 1 mm wide it is not considered significant. From a clinical standpoint though, whether 6 or 7 Q waves are present makes little difference.

Clinical Issues: The anterior wall is the most important of the three regions (anterior, inferior, and lateral) of the left ventricle and anterior wall myocardial infarctions are associated with increased risk of death and heart failure when compared to inferior wall and lateral wall myocardial infarctions.

Precordial ST Segment Elevation

Anterior Wall Myocardial Infarction (with Right Bundle Branch Block)

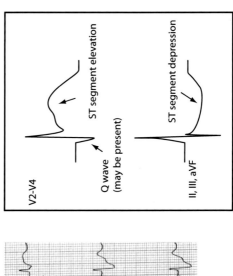

V2–V4

ST segment elevation

Q wave (may be present)

ST segment depression

II, III, aVF

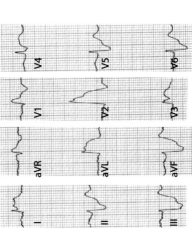

Figure 4.9:

Background: Conduction abnormalities may be seen in the setting of an anterior wall myocardial infarction. One of the earliest branches of the left anterior descending artery is the "first septal perforator" that "dives" into the septum and provides blood to the right bundle branch and the left anterior fascicle.

ECG: The ECG for this anterior wall myocardial infarction is different than the example in Figure 4.7. Both are associated with ST segment elevation in leads V_2 through V_4. In this example ST segment elevation is not present in the lateral precordium in leads V_5 and V_6 but prominent ST segment elevation is noted in I and aVL. Profound "reciprocal" ST segment depression is noted in the inferior leads (II, III, and aVF). The exact mechanism for reciprocal ST depression is not well understood, but from an ECG analysis standpoint the presence of "reciprocal" changes in the inferior leads is very strong evidence for cardiac injury. In this example abnormal Q waves are present in V_1 and V_2. The final

difference between Figures 4.7 and 4.8 is the QRS complex in V_1. In this example it is wide (0.16 s) and predominantly positive. This patient has right bundle branch block and left anterior fascicular block, problems that are introduced in Chapters 7 and 9. Compare this ECG and the ECG in Figure 4.7. Myocardial injury is associated with more prominent ST segment elevation, inferior reciprocal ST segment depression and Q waves. In fact, of all the ECG parameters, accompanying reciprocal ST depression is the best clue for deciding that ST segment elevation is due to myocardial injury.

Clinical Issues: As in Figure 4.7, the presence of an acute anterior wall myocardial infarction requires rapid identification and an attempt to restore blood flow to the myocardium at risk. In many cases this will involve transporting the patient to the catheterization laboratory for revascularization (angioplasty or stent) but could also require the use of powerful "clot buster" medications if necessary.

Precordial ST Segment Elevation

Anterior Wall Myocardial Infarction (with lateral extension)

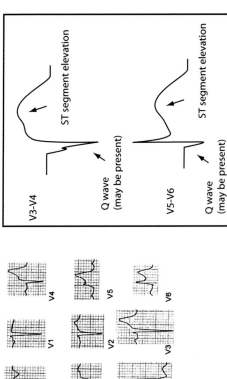

V3–V4

ST segment elevation

Q wave (may be present)

V5–V6

ST segment elevation

Q wave (may be present)

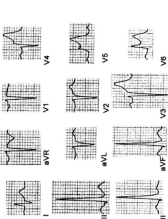

I
II
III
aVR
aVL
aVF
V1
V2
V3
V4
V5
V6

Figure 4.10:

Background: An anterolateral myocardial infarction can be due to occlusion of the left anterior descending, occlusion of a large diagonal branch, or a coronary artery that arises when the left anterior descending artery and the circumflex coronary artery branch. This artery is called a *ramus intermedius* and in this case instead of bifurcating the left main coronary artery trifurcates with the *ramus intermedius* forming the "middle tine of the fork."

ECG: In an anterolateral myocardial infarction ST segment elevation is usually not observed in V_1 and V_2 but rather extends more laterally to V_5 and in some cases V_6. In this example ST segment elevation is observed in V_3 through V_6 but the "high lateral" leads I and aVL do not have ST segment elevation. No reciprocal ST segment depression is present in this example and there are no Q waves. However, notice that there is no R wave even in lead V_4. This late transition is sometimes called "poor R wave progression" and is considered by some to be equivalent to a Q wave.

Clinical Issues: Again as in any STEMI, urgent attempts at reestablishing blood flow to the myocardium at risk are critical.

Precordial ST Segment Elevation

Anterior Wall Myocardial Infarction (LARGE with lateral extension)

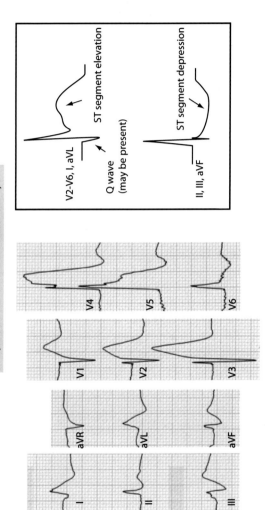

Figure 4.11:

Background: The specific leads with ST segment elevation will depend on the exact location of the blockage and the branches from the occluded artery. In general the more widespread the ST segment elevation, the more proximal ("upstream") the blockage, the more branches, and the larger the area at risk.

ECG: In this example marked ST segment elevation is observed in V_2 through V_5 and I and aVL. In particular, the ST segment elevation in V_4 is extremely prominent: The ST segment is 23 mm tall and taller than the QRS in that lead. Very prominent ST segment elevation is observed early during a myocardial infarction and has been given the name

"tombstones" by morbidly creative clinicians to emphasize the seriousness of this condition. Notice that since the ECG is recorded early in the myocardial infarction process the only abnormal Q wave is recorded in aVL and no Q waves are present in the precordial leads. Sometimes the ST segment can be hard to separate from the QRS complex. In this case the downsloping ST segment elevation in I and aVL could be mistaken as a widened QRS complex.

Clinical Issues: Patients with larger myocardial infarctions, if left untreated, have a very high future risk of sudden cardiac death and progressive heart failure.

Precordial ST Segment Elevation

Left Ventricular Aneurysm

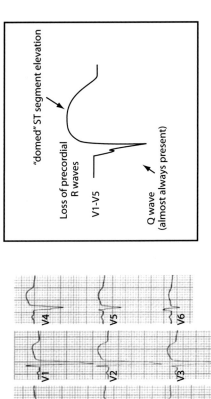

"domed" ST segment elevation

Loss of precordial R waves

V1–V5

Q wave (almost always present)

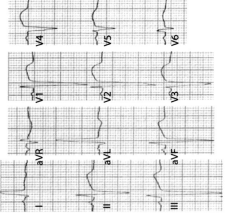

Figure 4.12:

Background: A left ventricular aneurysm is a defined area of the left ventricle that, instead of contracting, moves outward with systole. The most common cause of a left ventricular aneurysm is replacement of normal contracting myocardium with scar tissue due to a prior myocardial infarction. Anterior wall myocardial infarctions due to occlusion of the left anterior descending coronary artery are the most common cause of left ventricular aneurysms. The development of a left ventricular aneurysm after myocardial infarction is usually recognized 2–6 weeks after the acute event.

ECG: Persistent ST segment elevation in anterior leads that does not resolve in 2 weeks after a myocardial infarction should raise suspicion of a left ventricular aneurysm. The ST segment is elevation is dome shaped, accompanied by T wave inversion and Q waves and is most commonly observed in V_3 and V_4. Notice that unlike some of the examples of myocardial injury reciprocal ST segment changes are absent.

Clinical Issues: In general, ECG changes due to left ventricular aneurysm are identified by persistent ST segment changes and Q waves long after (weeks) any symptoms from the acute myocardial infarction have resolved. Patients with a left ventricular aneurysm are more susceptible to the development of congestive heart failure and ventricular arrhythmias. To reduce the likelihood of left ventricular aneurysm formation it is important to treat patients with drugs that lower blood pressues (angiotensin converting enzyme inhibitors) that will in turn reduce the amount of stress on the left ventricle (lower resistance that the heart must "pump against").

Precordial ST Segment Elevation

Apical Ballooning Syndrome

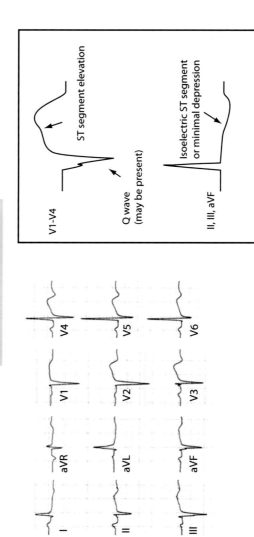

Figure 4.13:

Background: This is a syndrome (a syndrome is a collection of clinical findings that does not have a defined mechanism) of transient ballooning of the apical region of the left ventricle that is not associated with coronary artery occlusion. The apical ballooning is characterized by a thin neck with a large "outpouching" of the distal ventricle. It is more commonly observed in women who have experienced a sudden adrenergic surge. The name "Takotsubo" is derived from the Japanese word that means "octopus pot" that describes a narrow-necked vessel that is used to trap octopi (octopi can crawl into the pot but cannot get out).

ECG: Anterior ST segment elevation similar to occlusion of the LAD artery is observed. Q waves can also be present. Over time, the ECG will return to normal or near normal as the left ventricular function returns to normal. In this ECG upsloping ST segment elevation is observed in V_3–V_5.

Clinical Issues: There may be large areas of the apex that do not contract normally and cardiac enzymes may be elevated. Over time, left ventricular function and shape returns to normal. Patients that develop apical ballooning syndrome once are probably at higher risk of developing this problem again in settings associated with significant stress.

Precordial ST Segment Elevation

Hypertrophic Cardiomyopathy

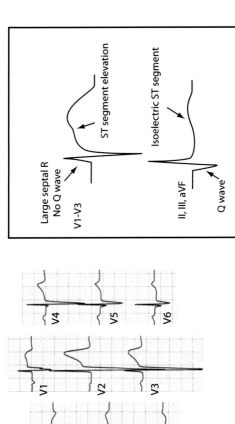

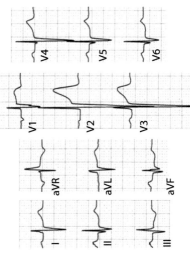

Figure 4.14:

Background: Hypertrophic cardiomyopathy is a hereditary disease characterized by abnormal thickening of the left ventricle. In most cases the thickening is generalized throughout the entire ventricle but in some cases the thickening is more prominent in specific regions such as the interventricular septum or the apex.

ECG: The ECG in hypertrophic cardiomyopathy can have many different presentations based on the location, extent, and magnitude of the left ventricular hypertrophy (Chapter 5, Figure 5.7). For the purposes of this discussion on ST segment changes, abnormal patterns of left ventricular depolarization can lead to anterior ST segment elevation.

The ST segment elevation is usually observed in leads with large QRS complexes and terminal S waves and is usually associated with prominent T waves (V_2 and V_3 in this example).

Clinical Issues: Most of the genetic abnormalities associated with hypertrophic cardiomyopathy are mutations that affect proteins of the sarcomere (the contractile unit within cardiac cells). Patients with hypertrophic cardiomyopathy can have shortness of breath due to inefficient filling of the left ventricle and pulmonary congestion. In addition, patients with hypertrophic cardiomyopathy are susceptible to ventricular arrhythmias and in some cases an implantable cardiac defibrillator (ICD) is required.

Precordial ST Segment Elevation

Brugada Syndrome "Sail"

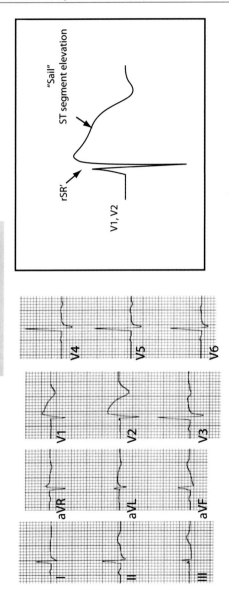

Figure 4.15:

Background: Another hereditary disease associated with anterior ST segment elevation is the Brugada Syndrome.

ECG: The ECG in the Brugada Syndrome has a characteristic appearance with a late positive deflection in the right precordial leads V_1 and V_2. In addition to the late positive deflection the ST segment will be elevated in these leads with a characteristic "sail" or "shark fin" pattern.

Clinical Issues: Patients with Brugada Syndrome are at higher risk for ventricular arrhythmias and sudden death.

Precordial ST Segment Elevation

Brugada Syndrome "Saddleback"

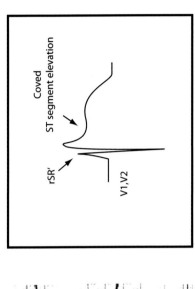

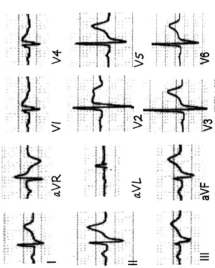

Figure 4.16:

Background: Another hereditary disease associated with anterior ST segment elevation is the Brugada Syndrome.

ECG: Another ECG pattern associated with the Brugada Syndrome has been described. The late terminal positive deflection (looks like right bundle branch block – Chapter 7, Figure 7.5) is present but the ST segment elevation has a sagging "saddleback" pattern.

Clinical Issues: Patients with Brugada Syndrome are at higher risk for ventricular arrhythmias and sudden death. Some studies suggest that the "saddleback" form has a better prognosis than the "shark fin" form.

Precordial ST Segment Elevation

Hyperkalemia

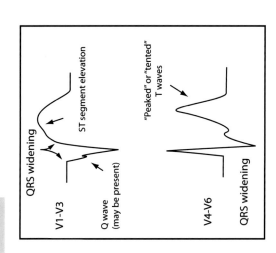

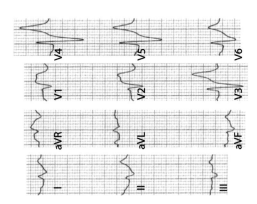

Figure 4.17:

Background: Any disease associated with renal failure can be associated with hyperkalemia.

ECG: The classic finding with hyperkalemia is peaked T waves (Chapter 6, Figure 6.3). However, hyperkalemia can also be associated with ST elevation and the development of Q waves and can sometimes be indistinguishable from an acute coronary artery occlusion. The only clue that can sometimes alert the clinician to hyperkalemia as the cause of ST segment elevation is the presence of peaked T waves in addition to the ST segment elevation. In the example ST segment elevation (impossible to distinguish from an anteroseptal myocardial infarction) but narrow based peaked T waves are present in the other anterior leads, particularly lead V_4. Importantly, hyperkalemia should not be associated with chest pain or other symptoms of myocardial ischemia. In patients with severe hyperkalemia patients will develop QRS widening often without a specific left or right bundle branch block pattern.

Clinical Issues: Hyperkalemia can be associated with life threatening arrhythmias and needs to be rapidly treated and the cause identified (usually renal failure). Hyperkalemia is treated with insulin and glucose (insulin 5–10 units and glucose 25 g (1 amp) intravenously), bicarbonate (44–88 mEq (1–2 amps) intravenously), and beta agonists (nebulized albuterol 10–20 mg) that quickly shift potassium to the intracellular space. In rare cases, intravenous calcium gluconate (10%, 5–30ml) or calcium chloride (5%, 5–30 ml) can be administered.

Precordial ST Segment Elevation (Lateral)

Lateral Myocardial Infarction

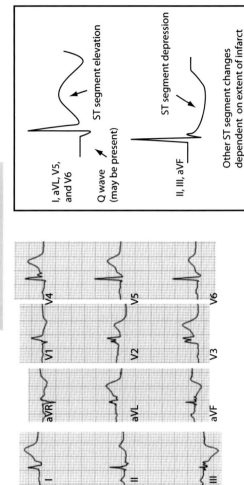

I, aVL, V5, and V6

ST segment elevation

Q wave (may be present)

II, III, aVF

ST segment depression

Other ST segment changes dependent on extent of infarct

Figure 4.18:

Background: The distinction between an anterolateral myocardial infarction and true lateral wall myocardial infarction may vary from interpreter to interpreter. Generally a lateral wall myocardial infarction is due to the occlusion of the circumflex coronary artery or one of its branches but can also be due to occlusion of a *ramus intermedius* or a diagonal branch from the left anterior descending artery if these arteries supply the lateral wall in an individual.

ECG: In a lateral myocardial wall myocardial infarction the ST segments will be elevated in leads I and aVL. Any accompanying ST segment elevation will depend on the vessel that is affected. In this example (compare to Figure 4.19), ST segment elevation is also observed in the precordial leads V_3 to V_6. Subtle reciprocal ST depression and T wave inversion is observed in the inferior leads (inverted T waves in leads III and aVF).

Clinical Issues: Lateral myocardial infarctions can be associated with significant occlusions in any of the three major coronary arteries depending on the patient's individual anatomy. The left anterior descending coronary artery has branches that plunge vertically into the interventricular septum (called septal perforators) and also course laterally toward the lateral apex (diagonal branches). Occlusion of a diagonal branch can cause a lateral myocardial infarction. The other main branch of the left main artery, the circumflex courses laterally between the left atrium and the left ventricle and occlusion of either the circumflex or its branches can cause a lateral myocardial infarction. As has been mentioned, some patients have a third branch, called a *ramus intermedius* that can be associated with a lateral wall myocardial infarction. Finally, in some patients the right coronary artery, after the posterior descending artery (which travels along the inferior portion of the interventricular septum toward the apex) branches off, will extend leftward and give rise to large posterolateral branches that supply blood to the lateral wall. Occlusion of one of these distal posterolateral branches can lead to a lateral myocardial infarction.

"Precordial" ST Segment Elevation (Lateral)

Lateral Myocardial Infarction (Only in I and aVL)

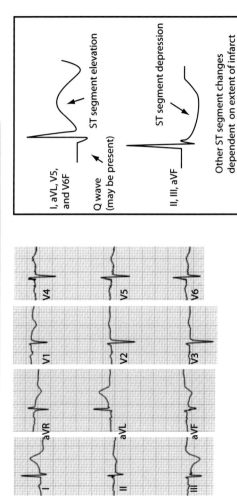

I, aVL, V5, and V6F — ST segment elevation

Q wave (may be present)

II, III, aVF — ST segment depression

Other ST segment changes dependent on extent of infarct

Figure 4.19:

Background: As described in Figure 4.18, lateral wall myocardial infarction can have many manifestations.

ECG: Given the significant patient variability for causes of lateral wall myocardial infarctions it is not surprising that the ECG manifestations also vary significantly. In this example, in addition to ST segment elevation is only present in the lateral leads I and aVL. The other lateral leads V_5 and V_6 do not have ST segment elevation. True lateral wall myocardial infarctions without involvement of other walls (anterorlateral or inferolateral) are almost always due to an occlusion in the circumflex coronary artery system (the circumflex itself or

one of its branches, the obtuse marginals). The diagnosis of a ST elevation due to a true lateral myocardial infarction can sometimes be difficult to make, but the presence of reciprocal changes in the inferior leads is an important clue that significant myocardial injury is present.

Clinical Issues: Again it is important to remember that the extent of ST segment elevation correlates roughly with the amount of myocardium that is at risk. However, since the lateral wall is "covered" by fewer leads than the anterior wall, estimating myocardium at risk can sometimes be difficult.

Precordial and Lateral ST Segment Elevation

Inferolateral Myocardial Infarction

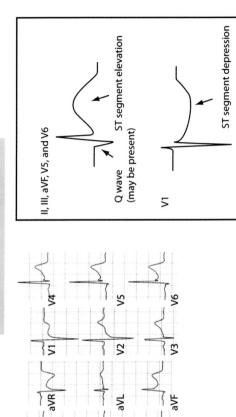

Figure 4.20:

Background: As discussed for the previous two figures, lateral myocardial infarction can be causes by lesions in any of the three major vasculature systems. This example is a lateral MI due to a right coronary artery lesion.

ECG: In this case ST segment elevation is prominent in the lateral leads with the addition of early repolarization (notice the "hooks" at the end of the QRS complex). In many myocardial infarctions that involve the lateral wall, the inferior ST segment elevation is most prominent in Lead II and less prominent in aVF and III. The presence of reciprocal ST depression in leads V_1 and V_2 is an important clue that acute myocardial injury is the cause for the extensive inferolateral ST segment elevation.

Clinical Issues: The same clinical problems as for the prior two figures.

Precordial and Lateral ST Segment Elevation

Pericarditis

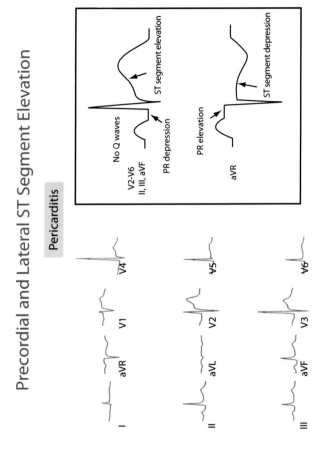

Figure 4.21:

Background: Pericarditis is the inflammation of the pericardium. Pericarditis can be observed in a number of conditions, most commonly after cardiac surgery. Other causes of pericarditis include viral, bacterial, and immunologic disorders. Most frequently no specific cause can be identified and the pericarditis is termed "idiopathic."

ECG: Classically, there are four stages of pericarditis that can evolve over a period of time that can vary from weeks to months. There are specific ventricular repolarization changes that occur in each stage:

Stage 1: Concave ST segment elevation
Stage 2: ST segment returns to baseline
Stage 3: T wave inversion
Stage 4: Gradual resolution of T waves.

The ST segment elevation generally is observed in the precordial leads and the inferior leads. Importantly there are no leads with reciprocal ST segment depression except for aVR. Pericarditis can also affect atrial tissue, so there will be PR segment depression best seen in the inferolateral leads and PR segment elevation in aVR. In comparison to the rest of the leads, lead aVR has as opposite response ST segment and PR response because it is the only ECG lead that "looks" at the heart from the right side and the inside surface of the heart. Since the pericardium overlies the heart, all of the leads except for aVR look "directly" at the injured pericardium resulting in widespread ST segment elevation. Lead aVR is probably the best lead for identifying pericarditis because of its characteristic presentation: PR segment elevation and the only lead with ST segment depression. The ST segment elevation has been described as "sagging" rather than the "domed" ST segment elevation observed in a STEMI.

Importantly in pericarditis ventricular depolarization will not be affected so Q waves will not be seen unless the patient has Q waves for another reason. The important teaching point is that Q waves associated with ST segment elevation are an important clue that myocardial injury is present. The ECG differences between pericarditis and an

Figure 4.21: (*Cont'd*)

inferolateral myocardial infarction are easily identified and are summarized in Table 4.2. Patients with pericarditis may develop significant atrial arrhythmias with atrial fibrillation as the most commonly observed abnormal rhythm.

Clinical Issues: One of the most common problems encountered in clinical medicine is evaluating the patient with chest pain. This is covered in detail in Chapter 14 but for the sake of this short discussion it is important to remember that since coronary arterial occlusion is potentially life-threatening and often has more significant long-term consequences than pericarditis, in general, possible coronary artery occlusion should always be the "working diagnosis" for any patient with chest pain.

Table 4.2: Pericarditis vs. Inferolateral Ischemia

ECG finding	Pericarditis	Inferolateral Ischemia
ST Segment elevation	• Inferolateral ST segment elevation	• Inferolateral ST segment elevation
ST Segment depression	• ST segment depression only in aVR	• Reciprocal ST segment depression in V1–V3
T waves	• No inverted T waves when the ST segment is elevated	• T waves may be inverted when the ST segment is elevated
PR segment	• PR segment elevation in aVR • PR segment depression in the inferolateral leads	• Isoelectric PR segment
QRS complex	• No Q waves	• Q waves may be present in the inferolateral leads

Inferior ST Segment Elevation

Normal variant

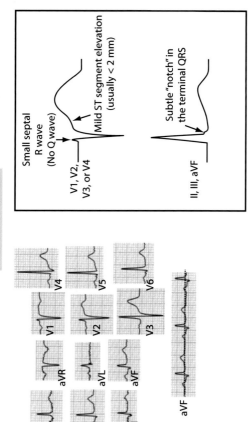

Small septal R wave (No Q wave)

V1, V2, V3, or V4

Mild ST segment elevation (usually < 2 mm)

Subtle "notch" in the terminal QRS

II, III, aVF

Figure 4.22:

Background: "Normal" ST segment elevation is normally most prominent in leads V_1 and V_2 although minor ST segment elevation may be seen in any lead particularly in the presence of early repolarization.

ECG: ST segment elevation less than or equal to 1 mm may be normally observed in any lead. In leads V_1 and V_2 where "normal" ST segment elevation is most commonly observed, ST segment elevation up to 2 mm is still within normal limits. It is important to evaluate any ST segment changes relative to the T-P segment. In this example, ST segment "elevation"

is most prominent in the inferior leads with the largest apparent deflection in lead aVF. Notice that when a horizontal line is drawn, the ST segment is actually reasonably isoelectric when compared to the T-P segment and the apparent ST depression is actually due to PR segment depression.

Clinical Issues: ECG findings must always be evaluated in the context of patient symptoms. However, evaluation of the ECG in a patient with early repolarization who is also complaining of chest pain, careful clinical evaluation is required.

Inferior ST Segment Elevation

Inferior Wall Myocardial Infarction

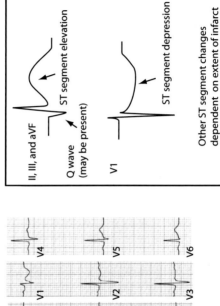

II, III, and aVF

ST segment elevation

Q wave
(may be present)

V1

ST segment depression

Other ST segment changes
dependent on extent of infarct

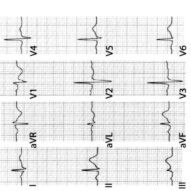

Figure 4.23:

Background: The posterior descending coronary artery travels along the interventricular groove parallel to the left anterior descending artery but on the most inferior portion of the heart and is most commonly a branch of the right coronary artery although in some cases it can arise from the circumflex coronary artery.

ECG: The hallmark of an inferior MI is inferior ST segment elevation. In this example the ST segment elevation is very subtle (compare it to Figure 4.19). Notice that the ST segment is elevated in relation to the T-P segment and that reciprocal ST segment depression is observed in lead aVL and V_1. In this example, Q waves in the inferior leads are not observed.

Clinical Issues: Inferior wall myocardial infarction in most cases is due to occlusion/stenosis of the right coronary artery. Generally patients with an inferior wall myocardial infarction have a better prognosis than those patients with an anterior wall myocardial infarction but in either case, steps aimed at reestablishing blood flow to the injured area is indicated.

Inferior ST Segment Elevation

Inferior Wall Myocardial Infarction (with first degree AV block)

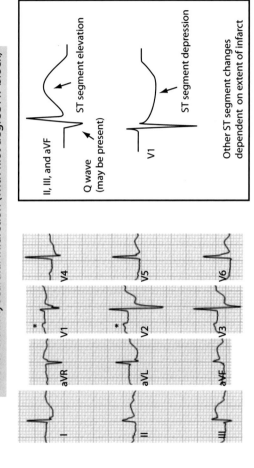

II, III, and aVF

ST segment elevation

Q wave
(may be present)

ST segment depression

V1

Other ST segment changes
dependent on extent of infarct

Figure 4.24:

Background: In any myocardial infarction there is evolution of ECG findings. In addition inferior wall myocardial infarction may be associated with atrioventricular (AV) block at least in part because the AV node receives its blood supply from the AV nodal branch from the right coronary artery.

ECG: The ECG will display different characteristics as the myocardial infarction "evolves" (Chapter 14, Figure 14.7). In this case the ST segments are elevated in the inferior leads and a Q wave is observed in lead III. Although Q waves may be observed in lead III under normal conditions, the presence of ST segment elevation with an accompanying Q wave should always arouse suspicion that the Q wave represents myocardial injury and abnormal ventricular depolarization. In the example the PR interval (the P wave is denoted by the *) is prolonged. Varying degrees of AV block can be observed during inferior wall myocardial infarction.

Clinical Issues: In general the AV conduction abnormalities associated with an inferior wall myocardial infarction resolve with time after the acute injury, but in some cases the recovery can be prolonged lasting weeks.

Inferior ST Segment Elevation

Inferior Wall Myocardial Infarction (Evolving)

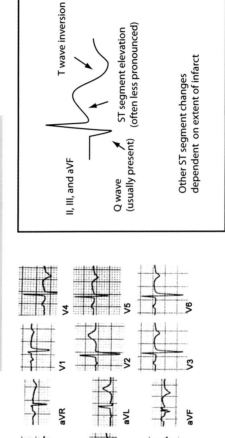

II, III, and aVF

T wave inversion

ST segment elevation
(often less pronounced)

Q wave
(usually present)

Other ST segment changes
dependent on extent of infarct

Figure 4.25:

Background: The evolution of ECG changes in an inferior wall myocardial infarction is fairly predictable but the timing of the progression of changes can be very variable.

ECG: In this example of an inferior wall myocardial infarction, Q waves due to abnormal ventricular depolarization are present in all three of the inferior leads (II, III, and aVF). The ST segments remain elevated in the inferior leads but the T waves are now inverted. In the setting of myocardial infarction, ST segment elevation is initially associated with upright T waves but after a variable amount of time (usually hours) the T waves become inverted while the ST segment remains elevated. In this example, abnormalities in V_5 and V_6 are also observed, probably due to large posterolateral branches that provide blood to the lower portion of the lateral wall of the left ventricle.

Clinical Issues: Although the presence of T wave inversion and Q waves suggests that initial occlusion of the artery occurred several hours ago, the primary treatment remains reestablishing adequate blood flow to the injured area.

Inferior ST Segment Elevation

Inferior Wall Myocardial Infarction ("Posterior" extension)

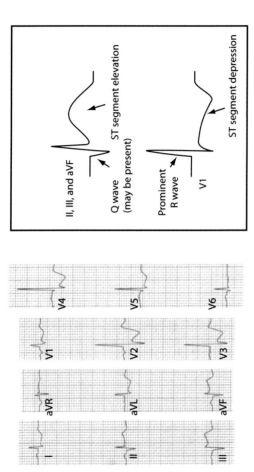

II, III, and aVF

ST segment elevation

Q wave
(may be present)

Prominent
R wave

V1

ST segment depression

Figure 4.26:

Background: After the posterior descending artery branches off to provide blood to the more apical regions of the inferior wall the right coronary artery often continues toward the lateral wall of the heart and may give off large posterolateral branches.

ECG: The larger posterolateral branches provide blood to the posterior wall. The posterior wall is commonly referred to in ECG texts although recent documents are trying to eliminate this word. Since there is no ECG lead that is directly over the "posterior" wall, injury and infarction in this area is usually assessed by evaluating lead V1 which is oriented 180° from the posterior wall. Since it is opposite, Q waves are manifest as a large R wave, ST segment elevation appears as ST depression, and an inverted T wave appears as an upright T wave. For these reasons the diagnosis of a "posterior" wall myocardial infarction is suggested by the presence of an R wave, ST segment depression, and an upright T wave in lead V_1.

Clinical Issues: The changes described for identifying a posterior wall myocardial infarction are generally late in the course of the myocardial infarction/injury but again management focuses on reestablishing blood flow to the abnormal region.

Inferior ST Segment Elevation

Inferior Wall Myocardial Infarction (With left bundle branch block)

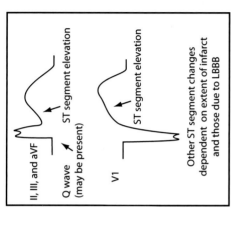

II, III, and aVF

Q wave
(may be present)

ST segment elevation

V1

ST segment elevation

Other ST segment changes
dependent on extent of infarct
and those due to LBBB

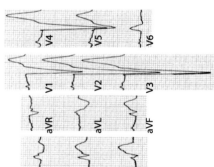

Figure 4.27:

Background: Evaluation of the ECG can be very difficult in left bundle branch block since both depolarization and repolarization are abnormal in the setting of left bundle branch block.

ECG: In general, left bundle branch block is associated with ST abnormalities that are "opposite" the direction of depolarization: A lead with a negative QRS complex will have ST segment elevation and a lead with a positive QRS complex will have ST segment depression. The presence of an ST segment change that is "concordant" with the QRS complex would be unexpected and may represent abnormal repolarization due to myocardial injury. In this example, abnormal ST segment elevation is observed in the inferior leads (since the QRS complexes are positive we would expect ST segment depression in these leads). In left bundle branch block, abnormal depolarization makes evaluation of depolarization abnormalities (Q waves) impossible.

Clinical Issues: The presence of left bundle branch block makes evaluation of the ECG for myocardial injury very problematic. For this reason, the clinician must depend almost exclusively on symptoms and physical examination findings.

Inferior ST Segment Elevation

Coronary artery spasm (right coronary artery)

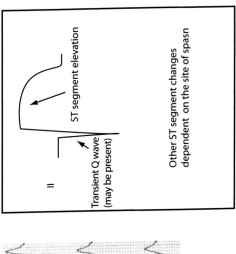

ST segment elevation

Transient Q wave
(may be present)

Other ST segment changes
dependent on the site of spasm

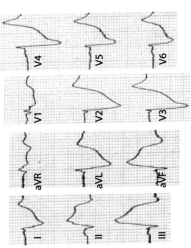

Figure 4.28:

Background: In addition to atherosclerosis and thrombus, another cause of myocardial injury/infarction is spasm of the coronary artery. The ECG changes are almost indistinguishable but often the ECG changes associated with spasm are more transient.

ECG: The ECG changes associated with coronary artery spasm are the same as for an acute myocardial infarction (not surprising since both lead to cessation of blood flow to an area of myocardium). In this case of spasm of the right

coronary artery, profound ST segment elevation is observed in the inferior leads with reciprocal ST segment depression in the anterior and lateral leads.

Clinical Issues: Generally coronary artery spasm resolves after several minutes and the ECG changes resolve as blood flow is reestablished. The treatment for spasm is generally medical therapy such as calcium channel blockers that promote vasodilation.

ST Segment Elevation in aVR

Critical Left Main

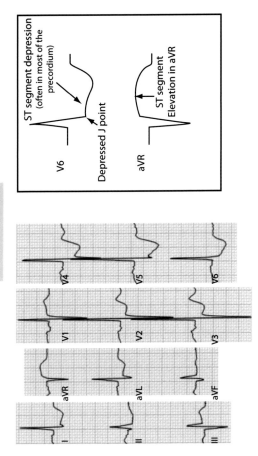

Figure 4.29: Left Main

Background: Although there are many anatomic variations, the left main coronary artery begins at the aorta and is usually about 1 to 2 cm long before it divides into the left anterior descending and circumflex coronary arteries. Occlusion of the left main coronary artery leads to large areas of myocardial injury and ischemia.

ECG: A critical left main coronary artery lesion often results in prominent ST segment depression in multiple leads. In the example, ST depression is observed in multiple leads: III, aVL and V_2 through V_6. ST segment elevation is observed in the leads that are oriented on the right of the heart: V_1, III, and aVR. In particular ST segment elevation is very prominent in aVR. In any patient with ST segment elevation in aVR, stenosis or a critical lesion in the left main coronary artery should be suspected. Lead aVR is the only lead that "looks"

directly at the endocardial surface ("inside") of the left ventricle. Since the endocardial surface is the most downstream area in the coronary artery circulation, limiting blood flow at the left main coronary artery leads to global ischemia that is most prominent on the endocardium.

Clinical Issues: Patients with a suspected lesion of the left main coronary artery require rapid and aggressive diagnostic and therapeutic management. In most cases an emergent cardiac catheterization to confirm the presence of a left main coronary artery lesion and to define the anatomy of the coronary arteries is performed. Although a percutaneous coronary artery angioplasty may be useful for managing the patient in the acute setting, ultimately coronary artery bypass grafting is often required.

CHAPTER 5

Abnormal Repolarization: ST Segment Depression

ST segment depression is also an important finding when evaluating the patient with chest pain. ST segment depression generally represents myocardial ischemia rather than myocardial injury. In this case, often a critical lesion is present, but some blood flow is reaching the endangered portions of the heart. Like ST segment elevation, ST segment depression can be observed in the anterior leads, the lateral leads, or the inferior leads. Unlike ST segment elevation, the location of ST segment depression does not correlate with the location of the myocardium at risk. For example, the presence of lateral ST segment depression can be due to significant lesions in the anterior descending, circumflex, or right coronary arteries. Isolated ST segment depression is most commonly observed in the lateral leads, but isolated inferior ST segment depression can also be observed. Isolated anterior ST segment depression is much less common (if anterior ST segment depression is observed, always check aVR for ST segment elevation and the possibility of a critical left main lesion or severe disease in all three coronary arteries (left anterior descending coronary artery, circumflex coronary artery, and right coronary artery) which some have called "left main equivalent").

The problem with using isolated ST segment depression as a specific sign for ischemia is that it may be present in some patients with left ventricular hypertrophy. High blood pressure or hypertension is an extremely common problem, with over 70% of people affected by age 70 years. Hypertension itself is not an issue; do you really feel the difference between a blood pressure of 140/90 and a blood pressure of 120/70? The problem is that hypertension causes damage to many organs including the heart, kidney, and brain. When contracting against higher pressures for an extended period of time, the heart responds by

ECG Interpretation for Everyone: An On-The-Spot Guide, First Edition.
Fred Kusumoto and Pam Bernath.
© 2012 John Wiley & Sons, Ltd. Published 2012 by John Wiley & Sons, Ltd.

Table 5.1: Factors determining whether abnormal ST segment depression is present and whether abnormal ST segment depression is more likely due to ischemia

---

Is abnormal ST segment depression present?
(Yes to any questions means abnormal)
- Is ST segment depression > 0.5 mm in V2 and V3, or > 1 mm in the other leads?
- Is the ST segment elevation present in two "adjacent" (contiguous) leads?

Is the abnormal ST segment depression due to myocardial injury?
(Yes to any questions means that myocardial ischemia is a likely cause)
- Is the ST depression new when compared to prior ECGs?
- Does the magnitude ST depression correlate with symptoms?
- Is the patient complaining of chest pain?
- Are Q waves present?

---

becoming larger and thicker. The larger and thicker heart leads to a characteristic set of changes that can be identified by ECG (Figure 5.6; Figures 8.12–8.14) but one of the changes is ST segment depression in the lateral leads. So here's the problem in a nutshell. Since hypertension is so common and some of these patients have left ventricular hypertrophy, if you were to evaluate 100 patients with ST segment depression the great majority would have lateral ST segment depression due to left ventricular hypertrophy rather than due to myocardial ischemia. In a patient complaining of chest pain, lateral ST segment depression becomes much more suspicious, particularly since hypertension is a risk factor for developing coronary artery disease. Clues for the evaluation of a patient with chest pain are summarized in Chapter 14.

ST segment depression is usually evaluated by determining the location of the J point, which is the point between the end of the QRS complex and the beginning of the ST segment. The threshold values for ST segment depression are the opposite of the threshold values for ST segment elevation. Since ST segment depression is extremely uncommon in V_2 and V_3, J point depression > 0.5 mm is considered significant, while J point depression > 1 mm is considered significant for the rest of the leads. The characteristics of abnormal ST depression and clues for identifying whether ST depression is due to myocardial ischemia are summarized in Table 5.1. The reader will note that often deciding whether ST depression is due to ischemia often depends on comparison between ECGs: New vs. old; presence or absence of symptoms.

ST segment depression

ST segment depression due to ischemia (with T wave inversion)

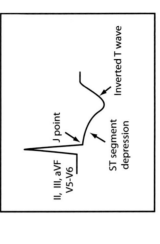

II, III, aVF
V5-V6

J point

ST segment depression

Inverted T wave

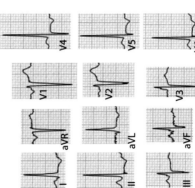

V1 V2 V3
aVR aVL aVF
I II III
V4 V5 V6

Figure 5.1:

Background: Inferolateral ST segment depression may be associated with ischemia. In fact the presence of ST segment depression is one of the important ECG criteria used for stress testing to identify ischemia.

ECG: ST segment depression due to inferolateral ischemia can have many manifestations. In this example there is horizontal ST depression associated with T wave inversion in leads II, V_5, and V_6. Abnormal T wave inversion is also present in I and aVL. The J point is the point where the QRS ends and the T wave begins and is where the magnitude of ST depression should be measured.

Clinical Issues: ST segment depression can be seen in a number of different conditions. As discussed in Chapter 14, fluctuation of the ST changes with waxing and waning of chest pain ("dynamic ECG changes") should raise concern that the ECG changes represent ischemia.

ST segment depression

ST segment depression due to ischemia (Upright T waves and Q waves)

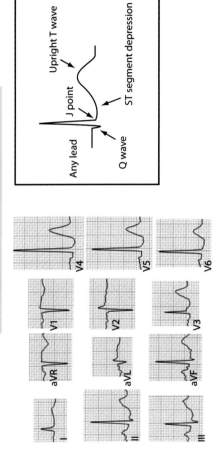

Any lead

Upright T wave

J point

ST segment depression

Q wave

Figure 5.2:

Background: ST depression is more likely due to ischemia if there is other evidence that coronary artery disease is present.

ECG: In this example ST depression is observed in the inferior leads, II, III, and aVF. Although the ST segments are "scooped" in the lateral leads the J point is only minimally depressed if at all. Unlike Figure 5.1, ST depression is not associated with changes in the T wave. In this example there are abnormal Q waves in V_1 and V_2. A Q wave is any initial negative wave. The Q wave in aVR is a normal finding since ventricular depolarization occurs from right to left. In addition Q waves in I and aVL may be seen in 30–40% of asymptomatic patients with no cardiac disease. However, the Q waves in two adjacent leads V_1 and V_2 are abnormal and suggest the possibility of a prior myocardial infarction. Evidence for prior myocardial infarction always increases the likelihood that the ST segment depression (and for that matter any associated repolarization changes) represents ischemia.

Clinical Issues: Again, if the patient is complaining of chest pain any ECG changes should be considered suspicious for ischemia.

ST segment depression

ST segment depression due to ischemia (critical left main stenosis)

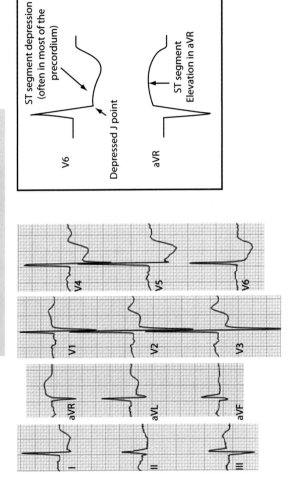

Figure 5.3:

Background: The left main coronary artery provides blood to most of the anterior wall and lateral wall of the left ventricle. Although left main coronary artery occlusion is associated with ST segment elevation in lead aVR (see Chapter 4, Figure 4.29), it is included here because the lateral ST depression is often extremely prominent and because of the severity of the problem.

ECG: The ECG in left main coronary artery occlusion is characterized by ST segment elevation in lead aVR but profound ST segment depression in the rest of the leads, particularly the anterolateral precordium (V_4 to V_6).

Clinical Issues: Patients with possible left main coronary artery lesions must be treated aggressively and usually require urgent cardiac catheterization to define the coronary artery anatomy.

ST segment depression

ST segment depression due to left bundle branch block

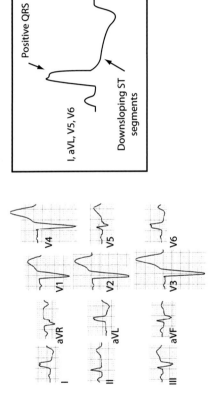

Figure 5.4:

Background: In the presence of left bundle branch block the ECG can be very difficult to interpret since ST segment changes are very common.

ECG: In general, in the presence of left bundle branch block, the ST segments will be elevated in the leads with a negative QRS complex and depressed in those leads with a positive QRS complex. For example in this case the downsloping ST segments and inverted T waves in I, aVL, and V_6 are all expected findings.

Clinical Issues: ST segment changes are extremely difficult to evaluate in the setting of bundle branch block, particularly in left bundle branch block.

ST segment depression

ST segment depression due to ischemia
(in the presence of left bundle branch block)

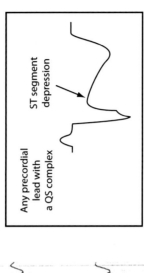

Any precordial
lead with
a QS complex

ST segment
depression

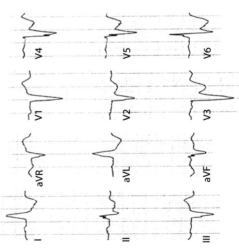

Figure 5.5:

Background: In the presence of left bundle branch block the ECG can be very difficult to interpret.

ECG: In general, in the presence of left bundle branch block, the ST segments will be elevated in the leads with a negative QRS complex and depressed in those leads with a positive QRS complex. The presence of ST segment depression in a lead with a negative QRS complex would be "unexpected" and should arouse suspicion for ischemia, particularly if the patient is complaining of chest pain. In the example, the ST segment depression in leads I and aVL would be expected since the QRS complex is positive; however, the ST segment depression in leads V_2 through V_5 is worrisome for ischemia since the QRS complex is negative.

Clinical Issues: In left bundle branch block, the presence of ST segment depression in a lead with a negative QRS complex should arouse suspicion if the patient is complaining of chest pain. The clinician should always remember the limitations of the ECG for evaluating ST segment changes in the setting of left bundle branch block.

ST segment depression

ST segment depression
due to left ventricular hypertrophy

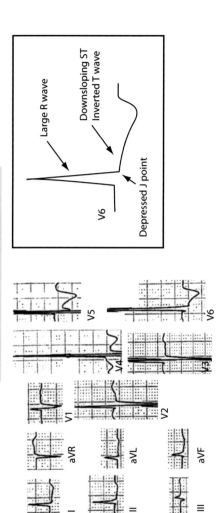

Figure 5.6:

Background: Left ventricular hypertrophy, usually due to hypertension, can be associated with repolarization changes and lateral ST segment depression.

ECG: The ST segment depression in left ventricular hypertrophy is usually downsloping. In this example, ST segment depression is noted in V5 and V6 and aVL. The key to identifying left ventricular hypertrophy as the cause of lateral ST segment depression generally includes identifying other ECG signs of left ventricular hypertrophy, including prominent QRS voltages in the lateral leads with large R waves and the presence of a biphasic P wave in lead V_1. In this case, the patient is in atrial fibrillation so P waves are not present.

Clinical Issues: The presence of left ventricular hypertrophy suggests that the left ventricle is contracting against a large afterload (systemic hypertension, aortic stenosis) that leads to a compensatory increase in left ventricular wall thickness.

ST segment depression

ST segment depression
due to hypertrophic cardiomyopathy

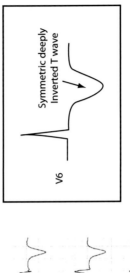

V6

Symmetric deeply
Inverted T wave

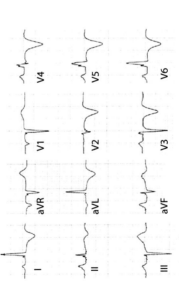

I

aVR

V1

V4

II

aVL

V2

V5

III

aVF

V3

V6

Figure 5.7:

Background: There are several different forms of hypertrophic cardiomyopathy (Chapter 4, Figure 4.14) that are classified by the location of the thickest region of the left ventricle. The most common form is generalized hypertrophy but sometimes the hypertrophy is disproportionately prominent in specific areas such as the septum or apex. The apical hypertrophy form is associated with lateral T wave inversion and may have ST segment depression.

ECG: Deep symmetric T wave inversion in V_5 and V_6 is characteristic and may be associated with mild ST segment depression (usually less than 1 mV).

Clinical Issues: Patients with apical hypertrophic cardiomyopathy may be asymptomatic or complain of shortness of breath due to the stiffer left ventricle and lung congestion due to increased left atrial and pulmonary venous pressures. Patients also are at higher risk for ventricular arrhythmias.

ST segment depression

ST segment depression due to digoxin

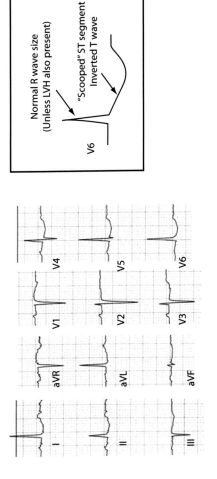

Normal R wave size
(Unless LVH also present)

"Scooped" ST segment
Inverted T wave

V6

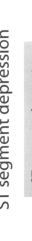

V4

V5

V6

V1

V2

V3

aVR

aVL

aVF

I

II

III

Figure 5.8:

Background: Digoxin is a drug that is used to control heart rate in patients with atrial fibrillation and now, much less commonly for the treatment of heart failure.

ECG: Although less commonly used today, digoxin is associated with characteristic ECG changes, in particular, downsloping of the lateral ST segments similar to what is observed in left ventricular hypertrophy but has a fairly characteristic "rounded" or "scooped" appearance. Notice that the J point itself is not depressed – rather there is "sagging" of the middle of the ST segment.

Clinical Issues: The ECG changes associated with digoxin are very commonly observed. Digoxin can be used in patients with heart failure, particularly if they also have atrial fibrillation.

CHAPTER 6

Abnormal Repolarization: T Wave Changes and the QT Interval

The ST segment correlates with the plateau phase of the ventricular action potential where all of the ventricular cells are depolarized and the voltages in the inside and outside of the cell are close to the same. However, over time the cell begins to repolarize and the voltage inside of the cell becomes negative compared to the outside. The T wave is produced as the ventricular cells repolarize. Think of the beginning of the T wave as the point where the first cells are repolarizing, the peak of the T wave when the greatest number of ventricular cells are repolarizing and the end of the T wave as the point when the last cells are repolarizing. As described in Chapter 2, repolarization occurs more gradually than depolarization, which leads to a "flatter" and more broad-based T wave. Since depolarization starts in the endocardium and repolarization starts in the epicardium, the normal "T wave follows the QRS complex."

In general, abnormal T waves are classified as either "peaked and prominent" or inverted. Inverted T waves are the most common T wave abnormality observed in clinical medicine. Identification of the cause of abnormal T waves can be extremely problematic because many medical problems can be associated with T wave inversion. Repolarization abnormalities follow a hierarchy of importance: ST segment elevation > ST segment depression > T wave inversion. For this reason, when evaluating ECGs look for ST elevation first, then ST segment depression, and only after isoelectric ST segments have been confirmed should you look for abnormal T waves.

Early repolarization is associated with ST segment elevation and prominent T waves, although in some cases the ST segment changes will be minimal. Peaked T waves can occur in two important abnormal

ECG Interpretation for Everyone: An On-The-Spot Guide, First Edition.
Fred Kusumoto and Pam Bernath.
© 2012 John Wiley & Sons, Ltd. Published 2012 by John Wiley & Sons, Ltd.

Table 6.1: Causes of QT interval prolongation

Etiology	Specific causes/issues
Hereditary	Long QT syndrome
Drug	Table 2
Metabolic	Hypokalemia
	Hypocalcemia
	Hypomagnesemia
	Hypothermia
Endocrine	Hypothyroidism
Central Nervous System	Subarachnoid hemorrhage

conditions. First peaked T waves can represent the first signs of injury to the heart and second, peaked T waves are usually described in the context of hyperkalemia. The two conditions can generally be separated electrocardiographically by the extent of the prominent T waves. In myocardial injury the peaked T waves are localized to a specific region supplied by the coronary artery while in hyperkalemia peaking of the T waves is more generalized.

Usually the direction of the QRS complex and the T wave are the same because depolarization and repolarization occur in opposite directions. From a practical standpoint, since ventricular depolarization occurs from right to left which leads to positive QRS complexes in aVL, I, II, and aVF in the frontal plane and V_4 through V_6 in the precordial plane, the T waves are positive in these leads in the setting of normal depolarization.

In addition to the shape of the T wave, the timing of the T wave relative to the QRS complex should be evaluated by measuring the QT interval. The QT interval is measured from the beginning of the QRS complex to the end of the T wave and provides a rough estimate of the duration of ventricular depolarization until the end of repolarization.

A prolonged QT interval can be observed under several conditions (Table 6.1). First, the QT interval can be prolonged because of a hereditary disorder called the Long QT Syndrome. Second, a number of drugs can cause QT interval prolongation (Table 6.2). Third, electrolyte disorders such as hypocalcemia and hypokalemia can cause QT interval prolongation.

Table 6.2: Drugs associated with QT interval prolongation

Drug Class	Specific Drugs
Antiarrhythmics	Amiodarone*
	Sotalol*
	Dofetilide*
	Ibutilide*
	Procainamide*
	Disopyramide*
Antihistamines	Terfenadine
Anti-infectives	Erythromycin
	Clarithromycin
	Pentamidine
Antimalarials	Chloroqiuine
Antipsychotics	Thioridazine*
	Chlorpromazine
	Haloperidol
Antidepressants	Amitryptyline
	Desipramine
	Imipramine
Opiates	Methadone
Other	Probucol
	Droperidol

* More likely to prolong the QT interval.

Prominent T waves

Early repolarization

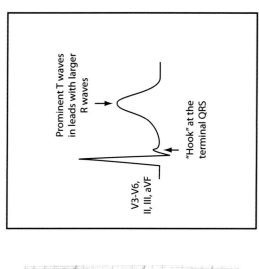

Prominent T waves in leads with larger R waves

"Hook" at the terminal QRS

V3-V6, II, III, aVF

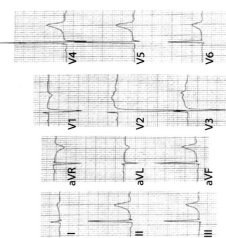

Figure 6.1:

Background: Patients with early repolarization will often have prominent T waves.

ECG: In early repolarization the prominent T waves will be observed in the inferolateral leads. Early repolarization should be suspected if there is the characteristic "hook" on the terminal portion of the QRS complex. In most cases, ST segment elevation will be observed in the leads with the most prominent T waves.

Clinical Issues: Early repolarization is fairly common, and is observed in about 7–12% of the general population. Interestingly, early repolarization may be more common in athletes with a prevalence of 30% in some studies.

Prominent T waves

Myocardial Injury

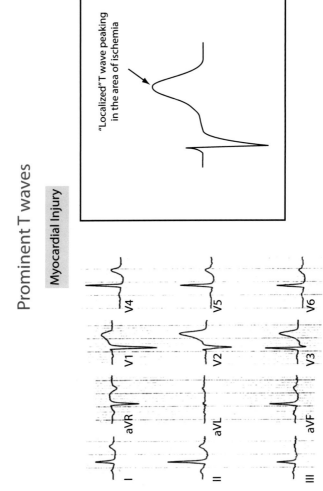

"Localized" T wave peaking in the area of ischemia

Figure 6.2:

Background: T wave peaking may be the first sign of myocardial injury on the ECG. Usually isolated T wave peaking is rapidly replaced by ST segment elevation (although the T waves remain prominent).

ECG: T wave peaking associated with myocardial injury is localized to a region supplied by a specific coronary artery and often, reciprocal ST segment changes are also observed. In the example, prominent T waves are noted in V_2 and V_3 due to a significant lesion in the left anterior descending coronary artery. In addition, notice the accompanying subtle ST segment depression in the lateral leads (V_4–V_6 and I) and the inferior leads (II and aVF).

Clinical Issues: The presence of localized T wave peaking is very suggestive of a significant coronary artery lesion and in the patient complaining of chest pain, serial ECGs and aggressive diagnostic evaluation is essential.

Prominent T waves

Hyperkalemia

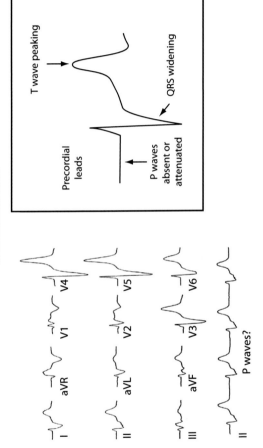

Figure 6.3:

Background: Generalized T wave peaking is the first sign of hyperkalemia. Peaking usually is observed when the serum K^+ is > 5.5 mM.

ECG: The first ECG sign in hyperkalemia is T waves peaking. If the hyperkalemia worsens (>6.5 mM) the QRS complex begins to widen and ST segment elevation may be observed (Chapter 4, Figure 4.17). In this example, prominent T waves are noted in V_3 through V_6 and leads II and I. In addition to the prominent T waves the QRS complex is wide without Q waves due to abnormal depolarization. With careful observation, ST segment elevation in leads V_1 and V_2 is also present. Finally, atrial tissue is more sensitive to hyperkalemia than ventricular tissue. This difference leads to loss of visible P wave activity particularly at extremely high K^+ levels (>8 mM). Interestingly the sinus node is still "driving" the heart and this condition is called a "sinoventricular" rhythm. Although it would be unusual for myocardial injury to have this combination of ECG changes, again the clinician must also take the patients symptoms into account. In hyperkalemia, chest pain is usually absent although patients may complain of nausea and generalized weakness.

Clinical Issues: Emergent treatment of hyperkalemia is reviewed in Chapter 4, Figure 4.17. In general once a blood sample is sent off, glucose and insulin are given. If the ECG changes are due to hyperkalemia, the ECG changes will rapidly improve.

T wave Inversion

Myocardial Ischemia

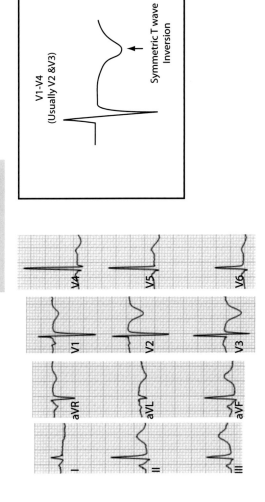

Figure 6.4:

Background: Ischemia may also cause T wave inversion.

ECG: T wave inversion is a very nonspecific finding particularly in the lateral leads because left ventricular hypertrophy is common. However, T wave inversion in V_3 and V_4 should arouse suspicion of ischemia in a patient with chest pain and has been associated with disease in the left anterior descending artery. The T wave inversion is usually symmetric and fairly prominent.

Clinical Issues: T wave inversion should arouse suspicion for ischemia in the patient with chest pain particularly if it is new when compared to prior ECGs.

T wave Inversion

Left ventricular hypertrophy

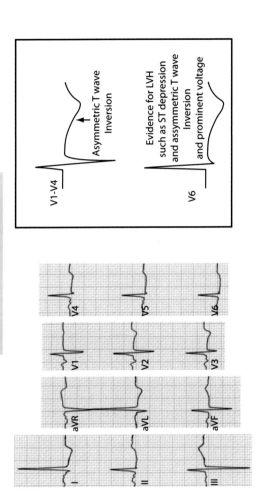

Abnormal Repolarization: T Wave Changes and the QT Interval **129**

Figure 6.5:

Background: Left ventricular hypertrophy can also cause anterior T wave inversion but is generally associated with accompanying lateral wall T wave inversion and ST segment depression.

ECG: In this example, inverted T waves are present in the entire precordium but notice that asymmetric downsloping ST segment depression is noted in the lateral leads I and aVL. The criteria for left ventricular hypertrophy are reviewed in detail in Chapter 8, Figures 8.12–14, but in general are characterized by large QRS complexes (due to increased left ventricular mass) and abnormal repolarization with ST depression and T wave inversion. Notice in this example the QRS in aVL is extremely large (approximately 20 mm).

Clinical Issues: The presence of repolarization abnormalities associated with left ventricular hypertrophy is associated with a worse prognosis in large population studies.

T wave Inversion

Arrhythmogenic right ventricular cardiomyopathy (ARVC)

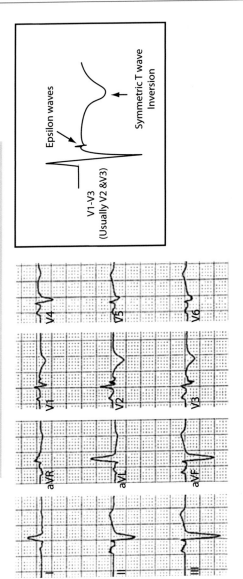

Figure 6.6:

Background: Arrhythmogenic right ventricular cardiomyopathy (ARVC) is a hereditary disease that leads to fatty infiltration of the right ventricle and is associated with the development of ventricular arrhythmias.

ECG: The ECG in ARVC has several characteristic findings. Anterior T wave inversion is present and is often associated with a right bundle branch block pattern (rSR' in V_1). In addition, in some cases discrete sharp "spikes" will be seen in the ST segment of leads V_1 and V_2. These are called epsilon waves and represent extremely late depolarization of a small part of the right ventricular outflow tract.

Clinical Issues: Patients with ARVC are at high risk for the development of ventricular arrhythmias and sudden cardiac death.

"Prolonged" QT

Apparent prolonged QT interval (prominent U wave)

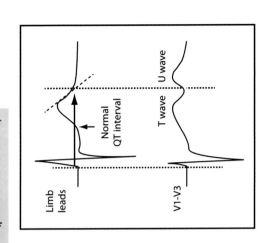

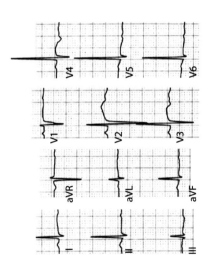

Figure 6.7:

Background: After the T wave, another deflection called the U wave can be observed.

ECG: The U wave is usually observed in young adults and is most commonly seen as a positive wave after the T wave in leads V_2 or V_3. The U wave is due to myocardial stretch rather than ventricular repolarization and for this reason most experts do not include the U wave in the measurement of the QT interval. The QT interval can be difficult to measure because the end of the T wave may be difficult to identify.

When calculating the QT interval, the steepest slope of the terminal downstroke or upstroke should be used to draw a "tangent." Where the tangent crosses the baseline should be used as the endpoint of the T wave. The QT interval must be corrected to rate to calculate the QTc (Chapter 3).

Clinical Issues: Accurate identification of patients with prolonged QT intervals is important because QT interval prolongation is associated with increased risk of ventricular arrhythmias and sudden cardiac death.

"Prolonged" QT

Apparent prolonged QT interval (prolonged PR interval)

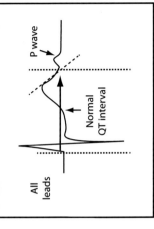

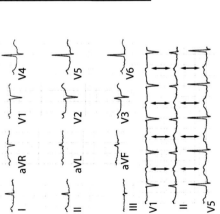

Figure 6.8:

Background: Sometimes the P wave will be mistaken as the terminal portion of the T wave.

ECG: In patients with significant disease of their AV node, PR interval prolongation may be observed (first degree AV block). In this example a prolonged PR interval leads to a P wave that occurs just after the T wave (double headed arrows). This situation can usually be identified by the apparent absence of a P wave in front of the QRS complex.

Clinical Issues: PR interval prolongation occurs when there is AV node disease that causes slower conduction through the AV node.

Prolonged QT

Long QT Syndrome

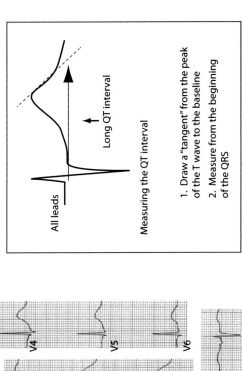

All leads

Measuring the QT interval

1. Draw a "tangent" from the peak of the T wave to the baseline

2. Measure from the beginning of the QRS

Long QT interval

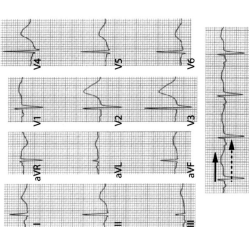

Figure 6.9:

Background: The Long QT Syndrome is a family of hereditary diseases associated with abnormalities in the ion channels responsible for repolarization.

ECG: There are many subtle ECG findings associated with the Long QT Syndrome but all are associated with prolongation of the QT interval. Delayed repolarization is often due to abnormal function of ion channels (particularly K^+ channels). On ECG the QT is prolonged. In general the QT interval (solid arrow) should be less than half the RR interval

(dashed arrow); in other words, you should be able to fit two QT intervals into one RR interval. The Long QT Syndrome is generally not associated with any QRS changes.

Clinical Issues: The Long QT Syndrome is associated with increased risk of ventricular arrhythmias. Prolongation of the action potential appears to reactivate the Na^+ and Ca^{2+} channels used for depolarization and lead to repetitive ventricular depolarization.

Prolonged QT

Drug (Ibutilide)

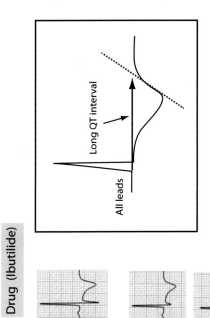

All leads

Long QT interval

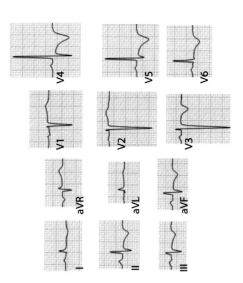

Figure 6.10:

Background: A number of drugs can cause QT interval prolongation (Table 6.2).

ECG: QT interval prolongation due to drugs may be associated with abnormal T waves such as lateral T wave inversion as in this case or may simply be due cause QT interval prolongation. In this case the anti-arrhythmic drug ibutilide led to a temporary increase in the QT interval.

Clinical Issues: Any cause of prolonged QT interval (hereditary, drugs, metabolic disorders, etc.) can be associated with the development of ventricular arrhythmias (Chapter 11, Figure 11.28). Anti-arrhythmic medications (particularly those that block K$^+$ channels) are the most common cause of QT interval prolongation.

Prolonged QT

Hypokalemia

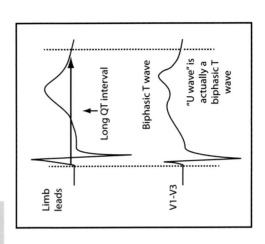

Limb leads

Long QT interval

Biphasic T wave

V1-V3

"U wave" is actually a biphasic T wave

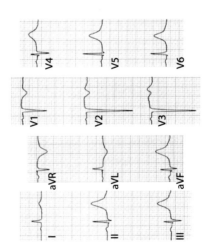

Figure 6.11:

Background: Hypokalemia can cause QT prolongation.

ECG: Traditionally QT prolongation due to a large "U wave" has been described as the classic sign for hypokalemia. More recent studies have shown that the "U wave" is actually a "double humped" or bifid T wave. The ECG changes associated with hypokalemia are more likely to be observed with progressive decreases in K^+. When the K^+ is between 3.0 and 3.5 mM, ECG changes will be observed in approximately 10% of people, while 80% of people will demonstrate ECG changes once the K^+ is <2.7 mM.

Clinical Issues: Hypokalemia requires careful replacement of K^+.

Prolonged QT

Hypocalcemia

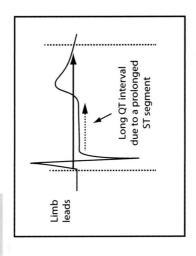

Limb leads

Long QT interval due to a prolonged ST segment

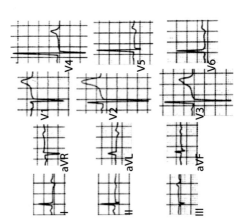

Figure 6.12:

Background: Hypocalcemia can cause QT interval prolongation.

ECG: The classic ECG change associated with hypocalcemia is prolongation of the ST segment with no change in the shape of the T wave.

Clinical Issues: The main treatment is correcting the low serum calcium with careful Ca^{2+} replacement.

Prolonged QT

Hypomagnesemia

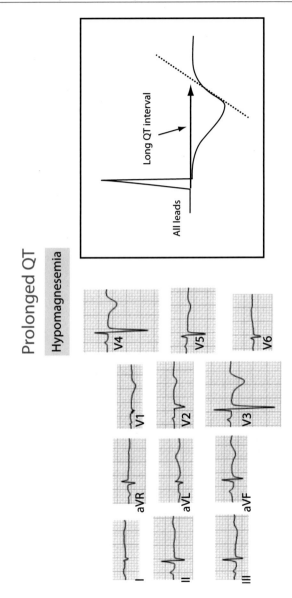

All leads

Long QT interval

Figure 6.13:

Background: Hypomagnesemia may be present in a variety of conditions including alchohol abuse and with medications, particularly diuretics.

ECG: Hypomagnesemia can also cause QT interval prolongation. The three electrolyte disorders have slightly different ECG manifestations. The QT interval prolongation due to hypokalemia is associated with a biphasic T wave. In hypocalcemia, QT interval prolongation is mainly due to ST segment prolongation. No specific ECG manifestations for hypomagnesemia have been described other than generalized prolongation of all components of the QT interval (ST segment and T wave) although some studies have suggested that hyopomagnesemia is associated with more prominent T waves. It should be noted that many patients will have several metabolic disorders, e.g. both hypokalemia and hypomagnesemia, so that specific ECG patterns other than a prolonged QT interval will be difficult to identify.

Clinical Issues: Generally, the treatment of hypomagnesemia is magnesium sulfate ($MgSO_4$), usually 1–3 grams given intravenously.

Prolonged QT

Subarachnoid hemmorhage

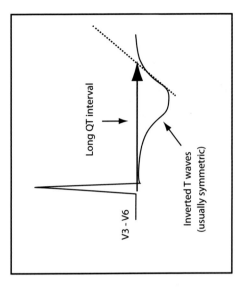

Long QT interval →

V3 - V6

Inverted T waves
(usually symmetric)

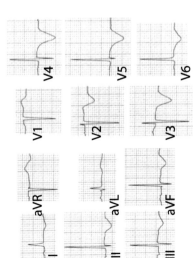

Figure 6.14:

Background: Subarachnoid hemorrhage can cause QT interval prolongation.

ECG: In subarachnoid hemorrhage, ECG changes may be observed in up to 80% of patients with QT prolongation with symmetric T wave inversion associated with bradycardia the characteristic finding. The specific mechanism for these ECG changes is not well understood although increased sympathetic and parasympathetic tone has been suggested.

Clinical Issues: The QT interval prolongation does not require specific treatment. The presence of ECG abnormalities does not affect prognosis.

CHAPTER 7

Abnormal Depolarization: A Prominent R Wave in V_1

So if you have gotten to this point you have finished evaluating the ST segment and the T wave. Remember that these two portions of the ECG represent ventricular repolarization. Since evaluation of patients with chest pain is one of the principal emergent clinical uses for the ECG, we have focused our initial discussion on ventricular repolarization. However, evaluation of ventricular depolarization is the other important component for evaluating ECG morphology (all the stuff other than rhythm), it is just that it can often be done at a more leisurely pace once active myocardial injury has been ruled out.

The easiest way to quickly assess ventricular depolarization is to examine lead V_1. The normal QRS is "narrow" (QRS < 0.12 s), and in lead V_1 the complex is usually characterized by an rS complex (Figure 7.1). With this in mind the two initial questions are: Is the QRS < 0.12 seconds? And is the QRS predominantly negative? If the answer to both of these questions is yes, the "general sequence and direction" of ventricular depolarization is probably normal. Once this has been established the ECG can be evaluated for frontal axis, Q waves, and other more subtle abnormalities of ventricular depolarization.

A narrow QRS is evidence that the ventricles are being activated simultaneously. However, if a wide QRS complex is present the ventricles are taking longer to depolarize because of relative delays in depolarization of some portions of the ventricles. The most common cause of a wide QRS complex is conduction block or delay in the left or right bundle (Figure 7.2). Block or delay in left bundle leads to depolarization of the right ventricle followed by depolarization in the left ventricle. Conversely, block or delay in the right bundle leads to initial left ventricular depolarization

ECG Interpretation for Everyone: An On-The-Spot Guide, First Edition.
Fred Kusumoto and Pam Bernath.
© 2012 John Wiley & Sons, Ltd. Published 2012 by John Wiley & Sons, Ltd.

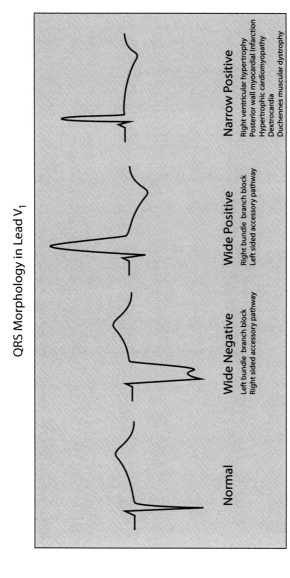

QRS Morphology in Lead V_1

Normal	Wide Negative	Wide Positive	Narrow Positive
	Left bundle branch block	Right bundle branch block	Right ventricular hypertrophy
	Right sided accessory pathway	Left sided accessory pathway	Posterior wall myocardial Infarction
			Hypertrophic cardiomyopathy
			Dextrocardia
			Duchennes muscular dystrophy

Figure 7.1:

Initial evaluation of ventricular depolarization is best done in lead V_1. The normal depolarization is "narrow and negative." With this in mind, abnormal depolarization can be "wide and negative," "narrow and positive," or "wide and positive."

Normal Depolarization

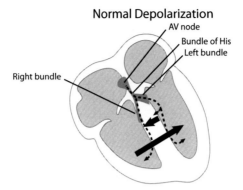

Right bundle branch block

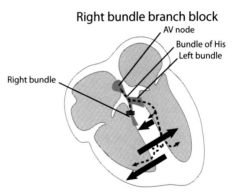

Left bundle branch block

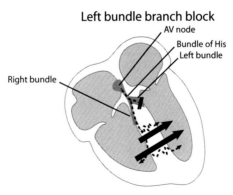

followed by right ventricular depolarization. Usually, because of its smaller mass, depolarization of the right ventricle is not observed on the ECG due to "canceling out" from depolarization of the larger left ventricle in the opposite direction. However, in right bundle branch block, depolarization of the right ventricle is late so it is "unopposed" (left ventricular depolarization has already occurred) and a late positive deflection (an R wave) is seen in V_1 and a corresponding late negative deflection (S wave) in V_6 (Figure 7.3). A much rarer cause of a wide QRS complex is *early* depolarization of a portion of the ventricles. Usually the AV node and His bundle form the only way for atrioventricular conduction because the valvular annulus (the fibrous rings that provide the structure for the valves) is electrically inert. In some patients the valvular annulus does not form completely and there is a residual thread of tissue called an accessory pathway that provides an additional electrical connection between the atria and the ventricles. In this case early depolarization of ventricular tissue near the insertion point leads to a wide QRS.

A predominantly negative QRS complex in lead V_1 means that ventricular depolarization is directed away from the right anterior chest (the location of V_1). This is the normally observed direction of depolarization because anatomically the left ventricle is located behind the right ventricle (Chapter 2, Figure 2.7). If the QRS is positive (a prominent R wave) in lead V_1, it means that a large portion of the ventricles is being depolarized from "back to front" (Figure 7.3). A "prominent R wave in V_1"

Figure 7.2:

This schematic shows ventricular depolarization (dotted arrows) and the resultant ECG forces (solid arrows) with normal ventricular depolarization, right bundle branch block, and left bundle branch block. During normal ventricular depolarization, after AV node and His bundle depolarization the septum is depolarized from left to right due to depolarization from the left bundle (shorter solid arrow). Near simultaneous depolarization of the left and right ventricles leads to a net leftward depolarization due to the larger left ventricular mass (longer solid arrow). In right bundle branch block, septal and left ventricular depolarization is unchanged but late depolarization of the right ventricle leads to a late rightward force. In left bundle branch block both the septal regions and the rest of the left ventricle are depolarized from right to left.

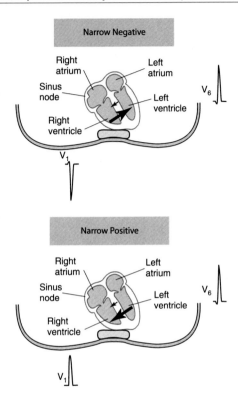

Figure 7.3:

The direction and timing of ventricular depolarization will change the QRS morphologies in V_1 and V_6. The easiest way to evaluate ventricular depolarization is to examine the QRS morphology in lead V_1 because this will give the clinician a sense for whether depolarization is directed toward the front of the chest or to the back. The most common cause of a wide negative QRS complex is left bundle branch block where there is sequential activation of the right ventricle followed by the left ventricle. The most common cause of a wide positive QRS complex is right bundle branch block where late depolarization of the right ventricles leads to a late positive wave (R') in lead V_1.

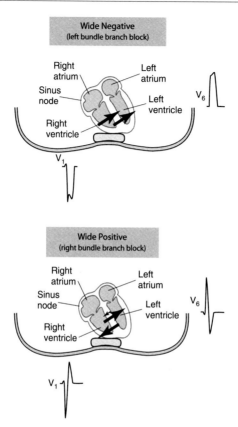

Figure 7.3: (*Cont'd*)

is most commonly due to right bundle branch block but is also observed in conditions that are associated with an increase in right ventricular size. However, right bundle branch block will always be characterized by a wide QRS. The common possible causes of a prominent R wave in V₁ are summarized in Figures 7.4 to 7.18.

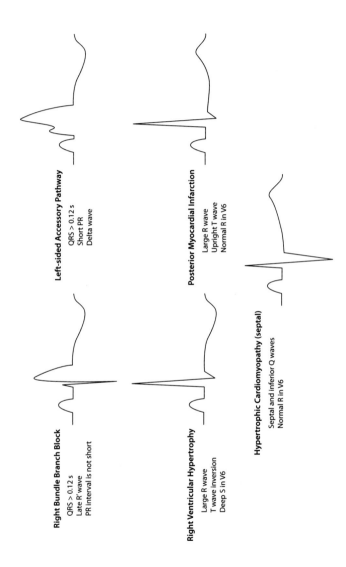

Right Bundle Branch Block

QRS > 0.12 s
Late R' wave
PR interval is not short

Left-sided Accessory Pathway

QRS > 0.12 s
Short PR
Delta wave

Right Ventricular Hypertrophy

Large R wave
T wave inversion
Deep S in V6

Posterior Myocardial Infarction

Large R wave
Upright T wave
Normal R in V6

Hypertrophic Cardiomyopathy (septal)

Septal and inferior Q waves
Normal R in V6

Figure 7.4:
There are several ECG clues that can help identify some of the common causes of a prominent R wave in V$_1$.

Prominent R Wave (Wide)

Right Bundle Branch Block

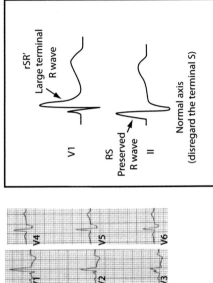

rSR'
Large terminal
R wave

V1

RS
Preserved
R wave

II

Normal axis
(disregard the terminal S)

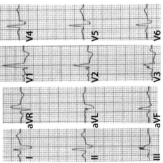

Figure 7.5:

Background: The most common cause of a prominent R wave in V$_1$ is the presence of right bundle branch block. Right bundle branch block may be observed in 1% of healthy populations and generally has no clinical consequence.

ECG: The ECG in right bundle branch block is characteristic. Late activation of the right ventricle leads to a late force directed anteriorly and toward the right chest (since this is where the right ventricle is located). This leads to a late positive R wave in lead V$_1$, and a late negative S wave in V$_6$ and an overall QRS width that is ≥ 0.12 s.

Clinical Issues: In general there are no additional clinical issues with right bundle branch block and no additional evaluation is required.

Prominent R Wave (Wide)

Right Bundle Branch Block (with Q waves)

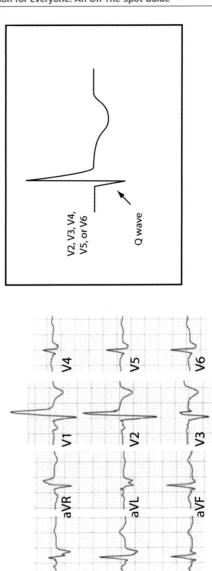

V2, V3, V4, V5, or V6

Q wave

Figure 7.6:

Background: As shown in Figure 7.2, initial septal activation is normal in right bundle branch block. As discussed in Chapter 8, one of the ECG signs of a myocardial infarction in the past is a Q wave or initial negative deflection in the QRS complex.

ECG: Since initial left ventricular activation is via the left bundle, in isolated right bundle branch block abnormal depolarization from a prior myocardial infarction may be observed. In the example, Q waves are present in leads V$_1$ and V$_2$. Remember that Q waves are simply an initial negative deflection in the QRS complex. Although initial negative deflections are expected in some leads such as aVR, in some cases they

are abnormal. In this case the Q waves represent a prior anteroseptal myocardial infarction. Remember that in these leads a small septal r wave would be normally observed. The loss of the septal r waves and the presence of the abnormal Q waves is due to a scar from the myocardial infarction that leads to a relative absence of electrical activity in these leads.

Clinical Issues: The presence of new abnormal Q waves should always arouse suspicion of a prior myocardial infarction. Many myocardial infarctions are "silent" either because of true absence of symptoms or, more likely, the patient thought chest pain was not due to a cardiac cause and did not seek medical attention.

Prominent R Wave (Wide)

Right Bundle Branch Block (with left anterior fascicular block)

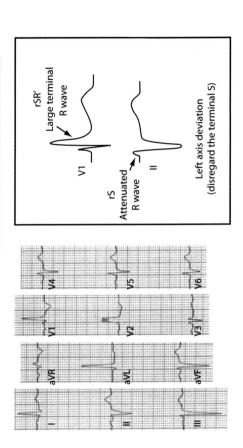

Figure 7.7:

Background: The left bundle divides into two major divisions: a left anterior fascicle and a left posterior fascicle. The right bundle is located adjacent to the left anterior fascicle and as a disease or degenerative process progresses right bundle branch block and left anterior fascicular block may occur together. Obviously if block occurs in the right bundle, and both divisions of the left bundle no atrioventricular conduction occurs (and a very slow heart rate – see Chapter 10).

ECG: In the setting of combined right bundle branch block and left anterior fasicular block, the left posterior bundle is providing initial ventricular activation. For this reason the right ventricle and the superior portion of the left ventricle are activated late. This leads not only to the characteristic findings of right bundle branch block but the ventricular axis in the frontal plane is directed upward.

Clinical Issues: When right bundle branch block and left anterior fascicular block are both present, the patient is dependent on the left posterior fascicle for ventricular activation. Fortunately the left posterior fascicular block is "short, fat, and stubby," so that it is generally fairly reliable and patients can do very well over extended periods of time with both right bundle branch block and left anterior fascicular block.

Prominent R Wave (Wide)

Right Bundle Branch Block (with left anterior fascicular block and a prolonged PR interval: "trifascicular block")

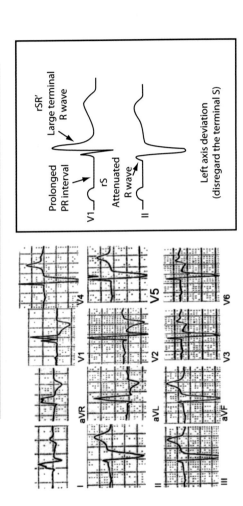

Figure 7.8:

Background: Evidence for extensive delays/block in the AV conduction system has often been called "trifascicular" block. Although this term has been used for many years, recent guidelines have discouraged its use since this term is often not accurate and has many ECG manifestations.

ECG: Trifascicular block is right bundle branch block and left anterior fascicular block combined with a prolonged PR interval. In the example a bizarre RBBB pattern is present in lead V$_1$, with an almost completely positive QRS complex and left anterior fascicular block (left axis deviation with the largest frontal plane R wave in aVL and aVL with a qR morphology). In addition, the PR interval is prolonged. Compare this ECG to the ECG in Figure 7.7.

Notice that the QRS is significantly wider (0.21 s) compared to Figure 7.7 (0.16 s).

Clinical Issues: As a general rule the wider the QRS complex the more severe the His Purkinje disease and myocardial disease. In fact several studies have shown a rough correlation between QRS width and left ventricular function: wider QRS complexes are associated with worse ejection fractions. Instead of using the term trifascicular block, it is better to simply understand that with more evidence for conduction tissue (AV node, His Bundle, and the bundle branches) disease such as accompanying fascicular block, prolongation of the PR interval, or QRS widening, the more likely that problems will arise in the future.

Prominent R Wave (Wide)

Accessory Pathway (WPW) (left lateral accessory pathway)

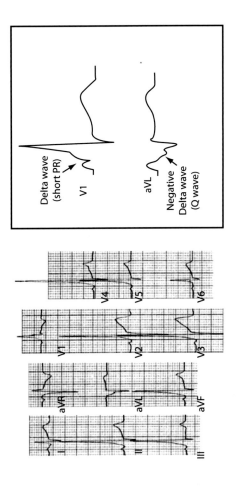

Delta wave (short PR)

V1

aVL

Negative Delta wave (Q wave)

Figure 7.9:

Background: Normally the AV node and His bundle form the only electrical connection between the atria and the ventricles because the annulus that forms the support for the mitral and tricuspid valves is electrically inert. In approximately 1/1,000 people there is another muscular connection (an accessory pathway) between the atria and ventricles because of incomplete formation of the valvular annulus. This condition is usually called the Wolff Parkinson White Syndrome to honor the three physicians that provided the most complete ECG description of this collection of findings in the 1920s.

ECG: Normally the AV node and His bundle are the sole source for ventricular depolarization but in the presence of an accessory pathway the ventricle can be depolarized from two sites so the QRS complex represents a "fusion" of activation between these two sources. Since most accessory pathways conduct rapidly relative to the AV node and His bundle, the PR interval is short and there is an initial "delta" wave due to activation via the accessory pathway. Remember that although AV node conduction is slow, depolarization is extremely rapid via the His Purkinje system so that in general the accessory pathway still activates a relatively small part of the ventricles even though it got a "head start." In patients with a left sided accessory pathway, since the left ventricle is located behind the right ventricle, this initial ventricular activation from the accessory pathway leads to a prominent R wave in V1. The best way to identify the presence of an accessory pathway is a short PR interval and an abnormal QRS complex due to the presence of the delta wave. In this example, the patient's accessory pathway is located in the lateral wall so the delta wave is negative (a q wave) in lead aVL.

Clinical Issues: Patients with accessory pathways are at higher risk for the development of abnormal fast heart rhythms (tachycardias or tachyarrhythmias). Normally since the AV node and His bundle form the only connection between the atria and ventricles, ventricular depolarization cannot affect subsequent atrial contraction (feedback). However with two connections between the atria and ventricles, it is possible that ventricular depolarization from the AV node could "echo" back to the atrium by depolarization of the accessory pathway.

Prominent R Wave (Wide)

Accessory Pathway (WPW) (left inferior accessory pathway)

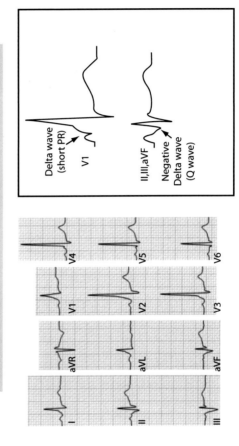

Delta wave (short PR)

V1

II,III,aVF

Negative Delta wave (Q wave)

Figure 7.10:

Background: An accessory pathway can be located in any spot between the atria and ventricles. The most common location for an accessory pathway is the left ventricle with the lateral wall a more common location than the inferior wall.

ECG: Regardless of the location of the accessory pathway the PR interval is generally short but the morphology of the QRS complex will depend on the location of the accessory pathways. Left sided accessory pathways cause positive R waves in V$_1$ and the specific location of the accessory pathway can be determined by the morphology of the delta wave. In general the delta wave will be negative in the leads that are located near the site of the accessory pathway

because initial ventricular depolarization radiates away from the accessory pathway. In this example, an accessory pathway in the inferior wall of the left ventricle will be associated with a negative delta wave in the inferior leads (II, III, and aVF).

Clinical Issues: The important findings on the ECG that are suggestive of an accessory pathway are a short PR interval and an abnormal QRS due to the presence of a delta wave. Accessory pathways located at the inferior wall of the heart (nearest to the diaphragm) have often been called posterior accessory pathways because they are located farthest away from the anterior chest using a cardiac surgeon's perspective.

"Prominent" R Wave (Narrow)

Normal septal R wave

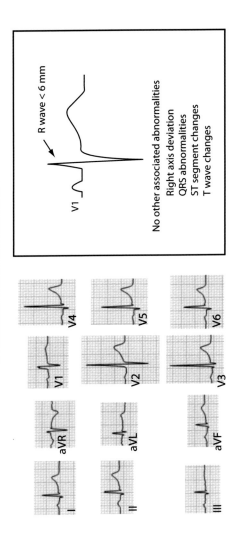

R wave < 6 mm

V1

No other associated abnormalities

Right axis deviation

QRS abnormalities

ST segment changes

T wave changes

Figure 7.11:

Background: A "septal" R wave up to 6 mm may be seen under normal conditions in V1. The R wave is more prominent in children. In fact, in newborns the R wave is often quite large because the right ventricle and left ventricle are pumping against similar "loads" (remember *in utero*, the lungs are not expanded and have a relatively high resistance). With aging, the R wave gradually decreases so that by the time someone is over 40 years old the R wave will be 1–2 mm with an upper range of 4–5 mm. Men have larger septal R waves than women.

ECG: As above an R wave <6 mm is normal in lead V_1, although an R wave >3–4 mm should be evaluated closely. In general a normal R wave can be identified by the "company it keeps" so it should not be associated with abnormal depolarization such as abnormal Q waves or axis deviation nor should there be associated repolarization changes such as ST segment deviation or abnormal T waves. As a corollary to the normal prominent R wave in V_1, while most individuals have a precordial transition zone where the R wave and S wave are equal at V_3 or V_4, about 2–6% of people will have a transition zone at V_1 and 12% of women and up to 25% of men will have a transition zone at V_2. In this example, the R wave is about 4 mm with a transition zone at V_1. The small inferolateral Q waves are from septal activation and are normal.

Clinical Uses: Obviously it is important to know the upper limits of normal for an R wave in V_1 and the normal precordial transition zone.

"Prominent" R Wave (Narrow)

Right intraventricular conduction delay (rSr' complex)

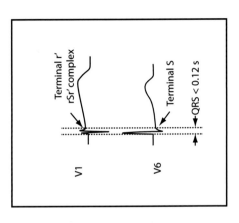

Terminal r'
rSr' complex

Terminal S

QRS < 0.12 s

V1

V6

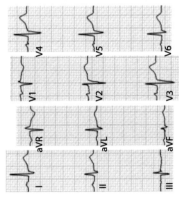

Figure 7.12:

Background: In some cases a small late r' will be observed in lead V$_1$ but the QRS will be < 0.12 s. In many cases this represents slightly delayed activation of the right ventricle (or relatively early normal activation of the left ventricle). This is generally a normal finding and is present in about 2–3% of healthy individuals.

ECG: Although not technically a "prominent R wave," it is convenient to talk about this ECG finding here because it has a similar mechanism as right bundle branch block. The ECG will have a rSr' signal with a normal QRS width with the r' < 5 mm and the r' wave will always be smaller than the S wave. Generally the accompanying frontal axis is normal. If there is accompanying frontal axis deviation (either left or right) the possibility of an atrial septal defect (a congenital "hole" between the left and right atria) should be considered. In the example, a late forward depolarization of the right ventricle leads to a small r' signal in lead V$_1$ and a corresponding small s wave in V$_6$. The patient has a slightly leftward but still normal frontal axis about 0° with the largest R wave recorded in lead I.

Clinical Issues: Generally there are no clinical conseqences from a right intraventricular conduction delay. However, the clinician should carefully exclude the presence of an atrial septal defect if significant left or right axis deviation is present (usually by physical examination and in some cases by echocardiography).

Prominent R Wave (Narrow)

Right ventricular hypertrophy

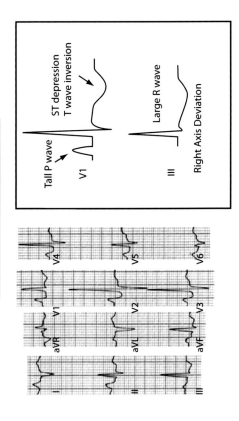

Figure 7.13:

Background: There are several conditions that are associated with right ventricular hypertrophy including lung diseases and congenital heart disease. Generally right ventricular hypertrophy develops in any condition in which the right ventricle must contract against higher pressures.

ECG: When significant right ventricular hypertrophy is present, if severe enough, the forces produced by right ventricular depolarization will be more prominent than the forces produced by left ventricular depolarization. This situation leads to a marked change in the direction of ventricular depolarization to left to right in the precordial plane and a rightward shift of the cardiac axis in the frontal plane. For this reason the hallmark of right ventricular hypertrophy is a prominent narrow R wave in lead V$_1$ and right axis deviation. In this example, right axis deviation is present with the largest R wave in the frontal leads recorded in lead III. The other important finding associated with right ventricular hypertrophy is also shown in this example: the prominent R wave with a normal QRS duration in lead V$_1$. Often in severe right ventricular hypertrophy the T wave will be inverted in lead V$_1$; in older textbooks this will often be called right

ventricular "strain." The rightward direction of precordial depolarization also leads to a deep S wave in lead V$_6$ as in this example where the S wave is larger than the R wave. Finally right ventricular hypertrophy will often lead to right atrial enlargement and the P wave will become more prominent. In this example notice how deeply negative the P wave is in aVR and very tall and "peaked" in lead V$_1$.

Clinical Issues: The presence of right ventricular hypertrophy by ECG is associated with significant disease. In fact, even though the left ventricle is responsible for pumping blood to the body and the right ventricle responsible for transporting blood to the lung, the presence of right ventricular hypertrophy has a far worse prognosis than left ventricular hypertrophy. In part this is because under normal conditions the pulmonary circulation offers very little resistance to flow. A useful analogy is to think of the pulmonary circulation as a large river delta, when flooding occurs upstream the delta easily accommodates the excess water. The development of right ventricular hypertrophy is a late event in most diseases and often heralds a very difficult future clinical course.

Prominent R Wave (Narrow)

Posterior wall myocardial infarction

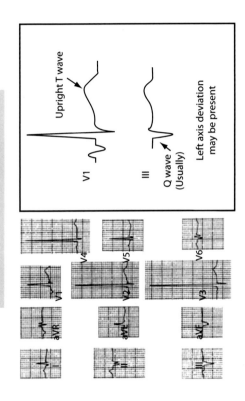

Upright T wave

V1

III

Q wave (Usually)

Left axis deviation may be present

V4 V5 V6
V1 V2 V3
aVR aVL aVF
I II III

Figure 7.14:

Background: The use of the term "posterior" myocardial infarction is no longer encouraged although it will still be frequently encountered in clinical medicine. The posterior wall was named because it was the wall farthest way from a surgeon looking at the heart from the front of the chest. In reference to the heart, this region is between/part of the inferior and lateral walls near the mitral annulus. Posterior infarction is usually due to occlusion of the right coronary artery or more rarely occlusion of the circumflex coronary artery.

ECG: Acute posterior wall myocardial infarction is discussed in Chapter 4 Figure 26 as there are usually associated ST changes. A posterior wall myocardial infarction that occurred in the past often does not have associated ST segment changes, rather the main finding is a prominent R wave in V$_1$ associated with an upright T wave. Remember that lead V$_1$ is directly opposite the posterior wall and the R wave and upright T wave actually represent an abnormal Q wave and T wave inversion if an electrode was placed directly over the injured area. Generally occlusion of the right coronary artery

causes an accompanying inferior wall myocardial infarction so Q waves in the inferior leads support the diagnosis of an old posterior wall myocardial infarction. In this example, the patient has both a posterior and an inferior wall myocardial infarction (inferior Qs in II, III, and aVF). The inferior wall myocardial infarction leads to left axis deviation with the largest R wave observed in aVL. Both a posterior accessory pathway and a posterior wall myocardial infarction will have a prominent R wave in V$_1$ associated with inferior Q waves. However, a posterior wall myocardial infarction can be differentiated from a left posterior accessory pathway because the PR interval will be normal and delta waves will not be seen. Since hypertension is a risk factor for coronary artery disease, in many cases, as in this example, an inverted or biphasic P wave will be observed in lead V$_1$.

Clinical Issues: The presence of an old posterior wall myocardial infarction requires the clinician to make sure that he or she is aggressively treating risk factors for coronary artery disease such as hypertension or high cholesterol.

Prominent R Wave (Narrow)

Dextrocardia

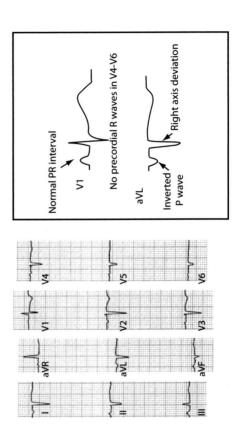

Normal PR interval

V1

No precordial R waves in V4–V6

aVL

Inverted P wave

Right axis deviation

Figure 7.15:

Background: Normally in the developing embryo, the heart forms on the left because of looping of the vascular tube. In some cases, the heart loops in the opposite direction leading to the heart located in the right chest or dextrocardia. Dextrocardia is rare and is present in less than 0.01% of the population.

ECG: In some cases of dextrocardia the heart is morphologically normal and the left ventricle is simply oriented to the right (this condition is usually associated with situs inversus where all of the organs are on the opposite side they are normally located). Dextrocardia leads to right axis deviation in the frontal leads, a prominent R wave in lead V$_1$, and S waves in the lateral leads (since ventricular activation is travelling away from the left side). When dextrocardia is associated with situs inversus, the sinus node is located to the left and the atria are activated from left to right. In this case the P wave is negative in aVL (rather than in aVR) although since the sinus node is still in the upper part of the right atrium the P waves are still upright in the inferior leads. In this example of dextrocardia the frontal axis is about −150° since the largest R wave is observed in aVR. The negative P wave and QS complex in aVL are the findings that with usual anatomy are found in aVR. Since the R wave is larger in V$_1$ compared to V$_2$, the precordial transition is in the right chest.

Clinical Issues: Generally there are no specific clinic issues associated with dextrocardia unless other cardiac abnormalities are present. When obtaining the ECG some recommend reversing the limb leads and placing the precordial leads in their usual position but in the right chest; if this is done the ECG will look relatively normal.

Prominent R Wave (Narrow)

Duchenne Muscular Dystrophy

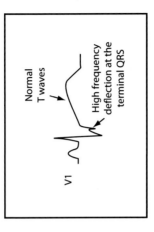

Normal T waves

High frequency deflection at the terminal QRS

V1

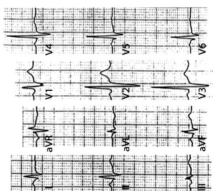

Figure 7.16:

Background: Duchenne muscular dystrophy is a hereditary disease that is due to a mutation in the gene that codes for dystrophin, a protein that is important for maintaining the cellular architecture in myocytes.

ECG: Duchenne muscular dystrophy leads to scarring of the posterior wall of the left ventricle leading to a prominent R wave in V$_1$ just as scarring from a posterior wall myocardial infarction causes a positive R wave in V$_1$. In addition, in some cases late activation of the posterior left ventricle will lead to a "spike" in the terminal portion of the QRS complex although this is a relatively uncommon finding. Now that

we have introduced some of the causes of a prominent R wave in V$_1$ we can see that an increased rightward force can be seen in two situations. First, conditions such as right ventricular hypertrophy and dextrocardia where there is larger mass to the right of the chest and second, conditions such as Duchenne muscular dystrophy or a posterior wall myocardial infarction in which there is loss of myocardial tissue in the posterior portion of the left ventricle.

Clinical Issues: Duchenne muscular dystrophy can be associated with heart failure in some cases due to progressive disease and also significant arrhythmias.

Prominent R Wave (Narrow)

Hypertrophic cardiomyopathy

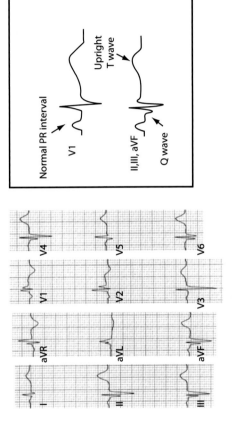

Figure 7.17:

Background: Hypertrophic cardiomyopathy is a genetic disorder due to mutations of proteins of the sarcomere (the actual structure that causes contraction).

ECG: In some cases the hypertrophic cardiomyopathy is most prominent in the left ventricular septum leading to a large initial left to right force that is also often oriented inferior to superior. This abnormal initial depolarization leads to a larger than expected septal r wave in V_1, a larger than expected septal q wave in V6, and abnormal Q waves in the inferior leads. Compare this ECG to the normal variant ECG (Figure 7.11). Q waves in the inferolateral leads are present in both, but in this case of hypertrophic cardiomyopathy the Q waves are extremely deep (4 mm; as will be discussed in

Chapter 8, abnormal Q waves are defined by lead, width, and depth) and there are associated ST segment elevation in leads V_1 and V_2, abnormal left axis deviation, and T wave inversion in aVL. Always remember to evaluate a prominent R wave in the context of the "company it keeps," so this R wave in V_1, although "normal" by voltage criteria, would be considered abnormal.

Clinical Issues: Hypertrophic cardiomyopathy can be associated with significant shortness of breath due to pulmonary congestion from elevated left atrial pressures due to a thickened stiff left ventricle. In addition, patients with hypertrophic cardiomyopathy are at higher risk for the development of ventricular arrhythmias.

Prominent R Wave (Wide)

Hypothermia (Osborn Wave)

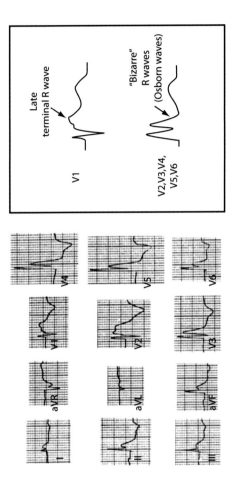

Late terminal R wave

V1

"Bizarre" R waves (Osborn waves)

V2, V3, V4, V5, V6

Figure 7.18:

Background: In severe cases of hypercalcemia and hypothermia, a distinctive bizarre late wave of depolarization can be observed that is often called an Osborn wave.

ECG: The Osborn wave is usually seen in the precordial leads as large late positive deflection just after the QRS complex. Since it coincides with the J point (remember our discussion of ST segment depression; the J point is the point between the end of the QRS and the beginning of the ST segment), the Osborn wave is also called a J wave. The Osborn wave becomes progressively more prominent as body temperature decreases and is seen very commonly when the body temperature is below 25° C. The specific cause of the Osborn wave has not been comprehensively studied but does appear to be mediated by abnormal function of K⁺ channels. In the leads where the Osborn wave is observed the T wave is usually inverted.

Clinical Issues: If an Osborn wave is present on the ECG, the underlying cause-hypothermia or hypercalcemia is generally easily identified.

Abnormal Depolarization: Wide QRS Complexes and Other Depolarization Abnormalities

Although a prominent R wave in lead V_1 is the easiest depolarization abnormality to quickly identify, obviously there are other QRS abnormalities that should be identified. If the QRS complex in lead V_1 is predominantly negative, the three remaining major parameters that have to be evaluated are: QRS width, frontal axis, identifying the presence of abnormal Q waves, and the overall size (voltage) of the QRS complex.

If the QRS is >0.12 seconds then the ventricles are not being activated simultaneously and it suggests that the two ventricles are not being depolarized by the His Purkinje system in the normal fashion. By far and away the most common cause of a wide QRS complex is abnormal conduction in either the right bundle or the left bundle. As discussed in Chapter 7, in right bundle branch block delayed activation of the right ventricle leads to a late positive force directed toward lead V1 and often results in a triphasic QRS in lead V_1 characterized by a large terminal R' wave.

In left bundle branch block, the septum is activated abnormally and more importantly the left ventricle is activated very late (Chapter 7, Figure 7.3). This results in a wide very negative QRS complex in lead V_1. A wide negative QRS complex is usually due to late activation of the lateral wall of the left ventricle due to left bundle branch block. Far rarer, a wide negative QRS complex in lead V_1 can be due to early depolarization of the right ventricle due to the presence of a right sided accessory pathway (Figure 8.1). Finally, another common cause of a wide negative QRS complex in lead V_1 is a pacemaker using a right ventricular lead.

ECG Interpretation for Everyone: An On-The-Spot Guide, First Edition.
Fred Kusumoto and Pam Bernath.
© 2012 John Wiley & Sons, Ltd. Published 2012 by John Wiley & Sons, Ltd.

Pacemakers are small, specialized computers/devices that transmit an electrical impulse to the heart via specialized leads. Pacemakers are typically used for the treatment of patients with slow heart rates.

Pacemakers are more comprehensively discussed in Chapter 12, but for this discussion it is important to note that most leads are placed in the right ventricle. With right ventricular pacing, ventricular depolarization travels from right to left and from front to back that does not utilize the

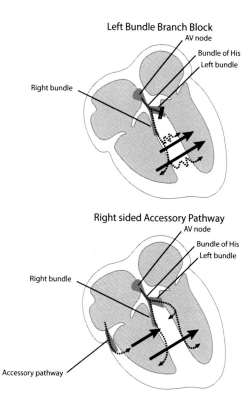

Figure 8.1:

Schematic showing the three most common causes of a wide negative QRS complex in lead V₁. As can be seen from the schematic, all three are associated with relatively late activation of the lateral wall of the left ventricle.

Right Ventricular Pacing

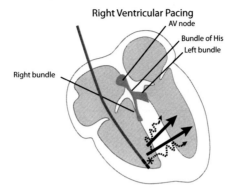

Figure 8.1: *(Cont'd)*

His Purkinje system. For this reason, right ventricular pacing is associated with a wide negative QRS complex.

Once you have established that the QRS is narrow and negative in V₁ the final things that need to be evaluated are the frontal axis, the presence of any abnormal Q waves, and the relative size of the QRS complex (Table 8.1). As described in Chapter 2, the frontal axis is generally from −35° to −110°. Left axis deviation is present if the axis is more negative (more leftward) than −35° and right axis deviation is present if the axis is more positive (more rightward) than 110°. The most common causes of left axis deviation are left ventricular hypertrophy and left anterior fascicular block. The most common causes of right axis deviation are left posterior fascicular block and right ventricular hypertrophy.

Q waves are any abnormal initial negative deflection in the QRS complex. A QS complex (thus a deep Q wave by definition) is expected in lead aVR and small q waves due to septal activation are expected in V₅ and V₆. Abnormal Q waves are "plump" (>0.04 s or 1 little box wide) and "deep" (>1 mV or 1 little box deep). Q waves can be observed in a number of conditions but where they have been historically important is for the identification of old myocardial infarctions. In a myocardial infarction, absence of depolarization in the affected area leads to net depolarization away from the affected region or a Q wave. Thus Q waves will be present in the leads that overly the affected area, so that in a patient with an old

Table 8.1: Evaluation of depolarization

Parameter	Specific ECG Question
QRS width	Is the QRS < 0.12 s?
QRS shape in V1	Is the QRS predominantly negative?
Frontal axis	Is the axis between −35° and 110°?
Q waves	Are abnormal Q waves absent?
QRS size (voltage)	Is the QRS voltage normal?

Any "No" answer is abnormal and the specific cause for the abnormal finding must be evaluated.

inferior wall myocardial infarction, Q waves will be present in leads II, III, and aVF. Q waves will also be present in I and aVL in left anterior fascicular block and in II, III, and aVF in left posterior fascicular block. Finally, a Q wave associated with an inverted T wave in lead III and an S wave in lead I has been called the S1Q3T3 pattern and has been linked to pulmonary embolus and right ventricular "strain" or "stress." It is important to keep in mind that abnormal Q waves can be seen in a variety of conditions and simply mean that ventricular depolarization is directed away from that specific lead.

The last depolarization abnormality to be evaluated is QRS size. As in the case of right ventricular hypertrophy, left ventricular hypertrophy leads to an increase in QRS size.

Wide Negative QRS in V1

Left Bundle Branch Block

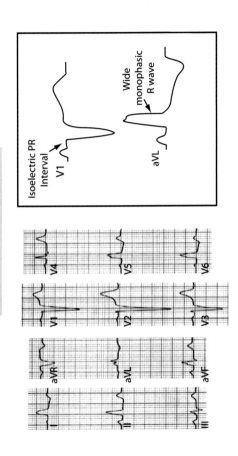

Isoelectric PR Interval

V1

Wide monophasic R wave

aVL

Figure 8.2:

Background: Left bundle branch block develops in about 1–2% of people who are followed for 20 years. In the United States left bundle branch block is associated with hypertension and coronary artery disease although worldwide the most common cause has been Chagas disease.

ECG: Left bundle branch block leads to abnormal activation of the septum and lateral wall and since the left ventricle is not activated over the His Purkinje system, the QRS is wide and deeply negative in lead V_1 and positive in lead V_6. Notice that left bundle branch block produces characteristic changes in repolarization even in the absence of ischemia. As a general guide, the ST segments and T waves will be in the opposite direction as the main QRS complex: Predominantly negative QRS complexes will be associated with upsloping ST segment elevation and upright T waves and predominantly positive QRS complexes will have downsloping ST segment depression and inverted T waves. Like many ECG "rules," this one also has many exceptions and should not be considered absolute; the upright T waves in lead II and the lateral leads I, V_5, and V_6 constitutes a normal finding. Compare this left bundle branch block ECG to the ECG in Chapter 5, Figure 5.4 where the T wave is inverted in aVL.

Clinical Issues: The left bundle branch is larger than the right bundle so that although isolated left bundle branch without any accompanying cardiac disease has not been associated with a worse prognosis in some large population studies, identification of left bundle branch block requires more detailed evaluation for any cardiac abnormalities.

Wide Negative QRS in V1

Right sided accessory pathway

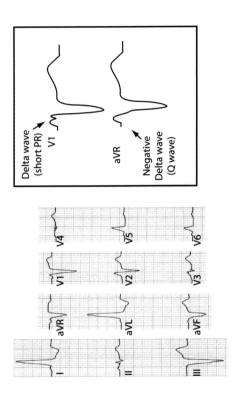

Figure 8.3:

Background: In the Wolff Parkinson White Syndrome, patients have an accessory pathway that connects the atria and ventricles (Chapter 7, Figures 7.9 and 7.10).

ECG: In patients with right sided accessory pathways, the right ventricle is activated first at the lateral wall of the tricuspid annulus. This leads to initial depolarization from right to left and a wide negative QS complex is observed in lead V_1 and a wide positive QRS complex (usually a monophasic R) in V6. Since the right ventricle is depolarized early, the PR interval is short. Depolarization of the ventricles in the Wolff Parkinson White Syndrome is from two sources- the accessory pathway and the AV node/His Purkinje system. The initial portion of the QRS complex is due to the accessory pathway and is usually called the delta wave. The shape of the delta wave provides a clue for the location of the accessory pathway. In right sided accessory pathways the delta wave is negative in lead aVR because initial ventricular depolarization is directed away from this lead.

Clinical Issues: Patients with the Wolff Parkinson White Syndrome are at higher risk for tachyarrhythmias.

Wide Negative QRS in V1

Right ventricular pacing

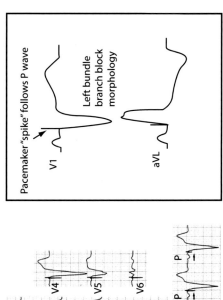

Pacemaker "spike" follows P wave

Left bundle branch block morphology

V1

aVL

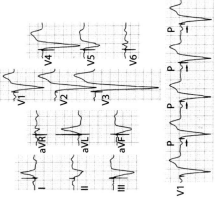

Figure 8.4:

Background: In many cases the only treatment for bradycardia is implantation of a permanent pacemaker. Since ventricular depolarization is critical for producing effective movement of blood to the systemic circulation a pacing lead in the ventricle is required. Ventricular pacing has traditionally been performed by placing a lead in the right ventricular apex since this chamber can be accessed from the large veins of the body (usually the large vein in the shoulder, and the lead is threaded through the superior *vena cava* through the right atrium and tricuspid valve to the right ventricle).

ECG: Ventricular pacing from the right ventricle provides a characteristic QRS complex. Since the right ventricle is activated first, the QRS complex usually has a left bundle branch morphology pattern (a monophasic QS complex in lead V_1). Ventricular pacing can be most easily differentiated from left bundle branch block by identifying the pacemaker spike (the electrical output that depolarized the ventricle). In addition since the pacing lead in often placed in the inferior portion of the right ventricular apex, since depolarization is activated away from the precordium and upward the QRS complexes are often negative in all of the precordial leads V_1 through V_6 and negative in the inferior leads. Left bundle branch block is not associated with negative QRS complexes in the inferior leads.

Clinical Issues: Pacing is more comprehensively covered in Chapter 12.

Q waves

Normal Q waves

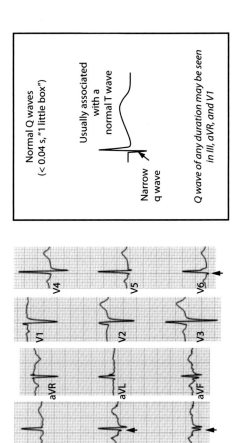

Normal Q waves
(< 0.04 s, "1 little box")

Usually associated
with a
normal T wave

Narrow
q wave

*Q wave of any duration may be seen
in III, aVR, and V1*

Figure 8.5:

Background: Small slender Q waves can be observed in some leads.

ECG: Normal Q waves usually are due to septal depolarization and are usually observed in the lateral precordial leads. Abnormal Q waves represent abnormal initial ventricular depolarization away from a specific lead and must be wider than 0.04 s or 1 "little" box to be considered significant. This criterion only refers to leads in which a Q wave would not be expected. Since ventricular depolarization occurs from right to left, Q waves are always present in aVR and may be observed in lead III. In fact since the identification of Q waves have always implied the presence of abnormal depolarization, traditionally the initial negative deflection in aVR is never referred to as a Q wave. In this example, the arrows show Q waves in leads II, III, and V6. The Q wave in III is a normal finding and would not be considered abnormal even though it is 0.04 s wide. The Q wave in lead II is not commonly observed but in this case is very narrow and small and is not pathologic. As mentioned earlier, the small q wave in V6 represents normal septal depolarization. A Q wave may also be observed in lead V_1 (remember it is contiguous to lead aVR) but any Q wave in lead V_2 is abnormal.

Clinical Issues: Normal Q waves are important to identify and may be confused with pathologic Q waves. In the end it is important to do a comprehensive evaluation in anyone with an "unexpected" Q wave. The differential diagnosis of Q waves is large and a more complete listing is provided in the Appendices (see Chapter 15, Table 15.2).

Q waves (Left Axis Deviation)

Left anterior fascicular block

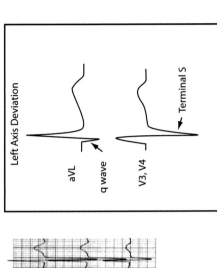

Left Axis Deviation

aVL

q wave

V3, V4

Terminal S

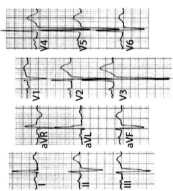

Figure 8.6:

Background: The left bundle divides into multiple branches but generally is considered to have two major branches:-a longer left anterior fascicle and a shorter thicker left posterior fascicle. A block in one of these fascicles will lead to characteristic ECG patterns because of the abnormal activation pattern of the left ventricle.

ECG: In left anterior fascicular block there is initial inferior depolarization of the left ventricle (from the left posterior fascicle) but the rest of the left ventricle-lateral wall and anterior wall is activated in an inferior to superior direction. This leads to a characteristic QRS pattern in the frontal leads with left axis deviation and qR complexes in leads I and aVL and rS complexes in the inferior leads. The initial inferiorly directed depolarization produces the small inferior q waves in the lateral leads and the small r waves in the inferior leads. The subsequent inferior to superior depolarization of the majority of the left ventricle leads to large R waves in the lateral leads and deep S waves in the inferior leads. The QRS axis is shifted leftward. Although both −30° and −45° have

been used as "cut-offs" for abnormal left axis deviation, it is important to remember that leftward (more superior) rotation of left ventricular depolarization represents a continuum. In other words although −45° is more abnormal than −30° block in the left anterior fascicle is probably not an "all or none" phenomenon. Like a tree, the left anterior fascicle has many branches and there will be progressively more superior rotation as more branches are lost. The QRS is widened slightly in left anterior fascicular block but since the left and right ventricles are activated simultaneously, the QRS complex is usually <0.12 s. In this example, the Q waves in I and aVL are less than 0.04 s and would not be considered abnormal.

Clinical Issues: Isolated left anterior fascicular block in and of itself is of no clinical consequence although one is always concerned that the process that caused the left anterior fascicular block is progressive. Left axis deviation is a common finding, an axis more leftward than −30° will be seen in 2–5% of asymptomatic men.

Q waves (Right Axis Deviation)

Left posterior fascicular block

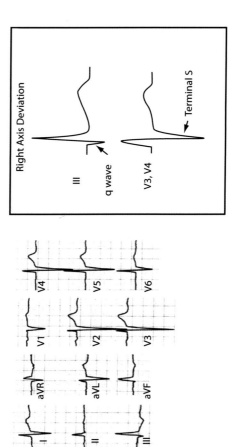

Figure 8.7:

Background: Probably based on its anatomy (short and stubby), left posterior fascicular block is far less common than left anterior fascicular block.

ECG: In left posterior fascicular block, initial activation of the ventricles is via the left anterior fascicle with initial activation of the anterior wall and with late activation of the inferior and lateral walls of the left ventricle. The ECG shows right axis deviation and qR complexes in the inferior leads and rS complexes in the lateral leads. Again, although an axis of 120° has been used as a "cut-off" for identifying abnormal right axis deviation, any axis more rightward than 90° should arouse suspicion. In the precordial leads, there is often a deep S wave in the anterior precordium due to depolarization directed away from the front of the chest. In this example, a Q waves are observed in lead III (normal finding) and aVF (< 0.04 s), but neither would be considered abnormal.

Clinical Issues: As in left anterior fascicular block, isolated left posterior fascicular block is generally not associated with any specific problems, but is much rarer.

Q waves (Abnormal)

Old lateral wall myocardial infarction

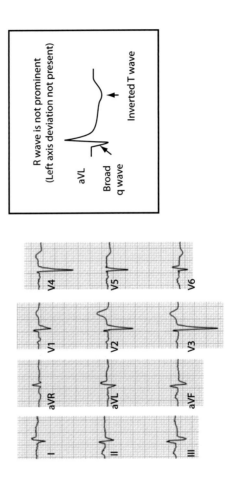

aVL

R wave is not prominent
(Left axis deviation not present)

Inverted T wave

Broad
q wave

Figure 8.8:

Background: The main reason for identifying abnormal Q waves is that they may represent a sign of an old myocardial infarction. The genesis of Q waves is complicated but they develop in leads that overly damaged myocardium. Scar and a relative reduction in depolarizing myocardial cells result in a net force of depolarization that appears to be directed away from the injured area.

ECG: Abnormal Q waves due to a prior myocardial infarction are generally present in regions that are supplied by a specific coronary artery or major branch. A lateral wall myocardial infarction may lead to abnormal Q waves in I, aVL, V_5 and V_6, while a prior inferior wall myocardial infarction may result in Q waves in the inferior leads (II, III, and aVF). In this example, abnormal Q waves are observed in I, aVL, V_5, and V_6. Q waves observed in I and aVL may be due to either left anterior fascicular block or a lateral wall

myocardial infarction. In a lateral wall myocardial infarction the axis will be normal or even rightward (due to loss of myocardium) and loss of R waves may be evident in the lateral precordial leads. In this example, there is no R wave in V_5 and even in V_6 where an R wave is present, the amplitude is extremely attenuated and the axis is extremely rightward with a predominantly positive QRS in aVR. Both of these findings are compelling evidence that the lateral Q waves are due to a prior myocardial infarction.

Clinical Issues: An old lateral wall myocardial infarction may be associated with heart failure and other symptoms. In particular, lateral wall contraction often provides support to the papillary muscle of the mitral valve. In some cases a lateral wall myocardial infarction can lead to the development of severe mitral regurgitation due to the loss of this support.

Q waves (Abnormal)

Old anterior wall myocardial infarction

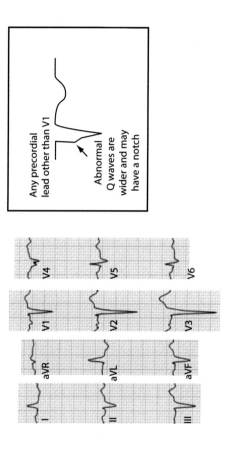

Any precordial lead other than V1

Abnormal Q waves are wider and may have a notch

Figure 8.9:

Background: Q waves may develop after an anterior wall myocardial infarction.

ECG: In this case, lead V_1 has a normal configuration with a small septal r wave. However, lead V_3 is markedly abnormal with a deep Q wave and absence of an R wave. Also notice that there is accompanying ST segment elevation. Notice that the precordial transition where the positive R wave is equal to the negative S wave is lead V_5 (or perhaps "V_4 and three quarters" since the R wave is slightly larger than the S). The normal R wave transition is V_2 through V_4 and some have described a late transition zone (V_5 or V_6) as "Poor R wave Progression." Poor R wave progression may be due to posterior rotation of the heart and can be seen in patients with left ventricular hypertrophy but can also be due to a relative loss of myocardial mass due to an old anterior wall myocardial infarction. Generally abnormal Q waves, like ST segment changes, are generally present in two contiguous leads. However, in this example, although there may be a small "nubbin" of an R wave in V_3 the extremely deep S wave is probably due to an anterior scar and is a Q wave "equivalent." In the anteroseptal leads the Q wave may be observed as a "notch" in the downstroke. The presence of a notch in the initial downstroke is strong evidence that an abnormal Q wave is present.

Clinical Issues: The presence of an anterior Q wave(s) should always spur additional evaluation.

Q waves (Abnormal)

Infiltrative disease (amyloidosis)

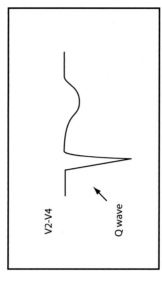

V2–V4

Q wave

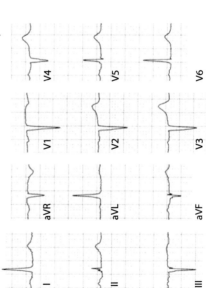

Figure 8.10:

Background: Although abnormal Q waves are most often due to a prior myocardial infarction, anterior Q waves may be observed in any condition that leads to loss of myocardium such as amyloidosis, sarcoidosis, or hemachromatosis.

ECG: In this example Q waves and accompanying loss of R waves is observed in the anterior leads V_2 through V_4. Again poor R wave progression is present with a precordial transition between V_4 and V_5. Although loss of R waves in the anterior precordium (often called "poor R wave progression") may be due to posterior rotation of the heart, the presence of a QS complex in lead V_4 is definitely abnormal. Often times, anterior Q waves in the setting of a prior myocardial infarction are associated with accompanying ST segment elevation due to the formation of a left ventricular aneurysm (Chapter 4, Figure 4.12). In this case the absence of accompanying ST segment elevation suggests an infiltrative disease as the cause for the ECG abnormalities. This patient had amyloidosis, where an abnormal protein called transthyretin is deposited in the heart with loss of myocytes.

Clinical Issues: By far and away the most common cause of anterior Q waves is coronary artery disease and an old prior myocardial infarction but may be due to other diseases that affect the ventricular myocardium.

Q waves (Abnormal?)

Pulmonary embolus (S1Q3T3)

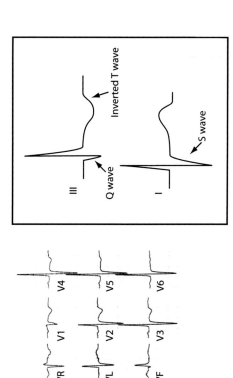

Figure 8.11:

Background: Pulmonary embolus is a common cause for the sudden development of chest pain. This diagnosis is generally made by tests other than the ECG.

ECG: The most common finding on ECG is simple increased heart rate due to generalized sympathetic activation in response to the hypoxia due to the pulmonary embolus. One ECG pattern that has been associated with pulmonary embolus is the S1Q3T3 pattern that is characterized by an S wave in lead I, and a Q wave and an inverted T wave in lead III. The depolarization pattern is thought to be due to a more rightward orientation of the frontal axis. The T wave inversion is thought to be due to hypoxia. In this example of a patient with a proven large pulmonary embolus, a deep S wave is noted in I, and a deep Q wave in lead III. The T wave is upright but there is some very subtle ST segment depression.

Clinical Issues: Pulmonary embolus (usually due to a blood clot that has broken off from a clot in the leg and traveled to the pulmonary arteries) should be in the differential diagnosis of anyone complaining of sudden onset of chest pain particularly with associated shortness of breath. Although the S1Q3T3 pattern is more commonly observed in pulmonary embolus and should arouse suspicion if present, in general the ECG has very little, if any, use for the identification of pulmonary embolus.

Prominent Voltage

Left ventricular hypertrophy (aVL)

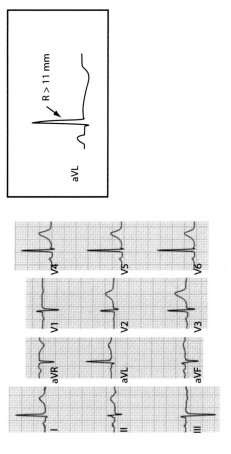

Figure 8.12:

Background: One of the principal problems associated with hypertension is the development of left ventricular hypertrophy. Thickening of the left ventricle is a way for the heart to respond to contracting against higher pressures (also called higher afterload) in hypertension.

ECG: Left ventricular hypertrophy is associated with both depolarization and repolarization changes. Since the left ventricle is larger and thicker, the voltages measured on the ECG are usually larger. Abnormal depolarization leads to abnormal repolarization most often associated with lateral ST depression and T wave inversion. One of the oldest criteria for left ventricular hypertrophy is an R wave >11 mm in lead aVL, as shown in this example.

Clinical Issues: Identification of ECG criteria for left ventricular hypertrophy should spur further cardiac evaluation. Often an echocardiogram is required to evaluate the severity of left ventricular hypertrophy and rule out any valvular causes of left ventricular hypertrophy, such as aortic valve stenosis.

Prominent Voltage

Left ventricular hypertrophy (V1, V6)

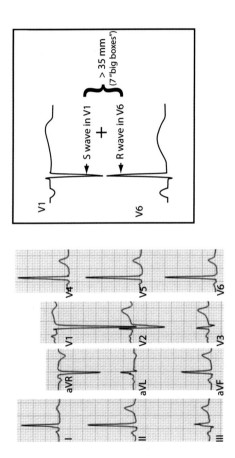

Figure 8.13:

Background: Since identification of left ventricular hypertrophy can be an important clinical issue, several different criteria for identification of left ventricular hypertrophy have been developed.

ECG: In addition to a large R wave in aVL, large voltages in the precordial leads have also been used as criteria for identification of left ventricular hypertrophy. If the sum of the voltage of the S wave in V_1 and the R wave in V_6 is > 35 mm, left ventricular hypertrophy is present.

Clinical Issues: The presence of left ventricular hypertrophy by ECG in a patient with hypertension is evidence that the hypertension is significant and probably has not been optimally controlled.

Prominent Voltage

Left ventricular hypertrophy (Romhilt-Estes)

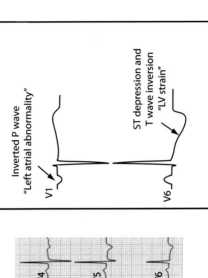

Inverted P wave
"Left atrial abnormality"

V1

ST depression and
T wave inversion
"LV strain"

V6

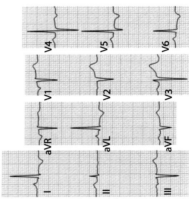

I

II

III

aVR

aVL

aVF

V1

V2

V3

V4

V5

V6

Figure 8.14:

Background: In addition to increased voltage due to increased left ventricular size and thickness, the presence of repolarization changes and other indirect evidence for left ventricular hypertrophy have also been used to identify left ventricular hypertrophy.

ECG: In an effort to increase the ability of the ECG to identify patients with left ventricular hypertrophy, some methods use a combination of different ECG findings together. In the most commonly used system, named the Romhilt Estes criteria for the two investigators who initially described the method, points are awarded for different findings. Although QRS voltage is used, points are also given for the presence of repolarization abnormalities (ST depression and T wave inversion) or a left atrial abnormality. The presence of left atrial abnormality suggests that the left atrium has enlarged/thickened in response to contracting against a thick left ventricle. The Romhilt Estes point system is summarized in in the Appendices (see Table 15.4). It is difficult to remember all of the points for each of the specific ECG findings but from a practical standpoint, a patient has left ventricular hypertrophy if both left atrial abnormality and repolarization abnormalities are present.

CHAPTER 9

Arrhythmias: Normal Rates and Skips

Arrhythmias are classified by their rate (Figure 9.1). Abnormally slow heart rhythms are called bradycardias from the Greek root "brady," which means slow. Chapter 10 provides a comprehensive discussion of bradycardia. Abnormally fast hearts are called tachycardias from the Greek root "tachy," which means "fast" and are covered in Chapter 11 (good luck when you come to this chapter, this is the most complicated of the arrhythmia topics). In between these two extremes are a diverse collection of arrhythmias with normal heart rates that will be the subject of this chapter.

We discussed normal rhythm in Chapter 3, Figure 3.4. In a normal rhythm the sinus node is generating the cardiac impulse and initiating atrial depolarization and every atrial depolarization is followed by a timely ventricular depolarization. The source of atrial depolarization is identified by examining the shape of the P wave. Since the sinus node is located at the superior *vena cava*/right atrial junction, it is positive in lead II and negative in aVR. If the AV node and His bundle are conducting normally, ventricular depolarization (a QRS complex) will follow the P wave. With normal conduction through the AV node and His bundle, the PR interval (the interval measured from the beginning of the P wave to the beginning of the QRS complex) will be < 0.20 s.

If the patient is having an abnormal heart rhythm (arrhythmia) at a normal rate there are two basic questions that must be answered. First, is the basic rhythm being generated by the sinus node? Second, are there irregular heart beats?

ECG Interpretation for Everyone: An On-The-Spot Guide, First Edition.
Fred Kusumoto and Pam Bernath.
© 2012 John Wiley & Sons, Ltd. Published 2012 by John Wiley & Sons, Ltd.

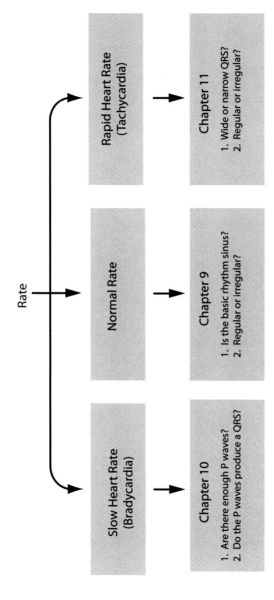

Figure 9.1: The basic algorithm for abnormal heart rhythms (arrhythmias).

Regular Rhythm

Normal Sinus Rhythm

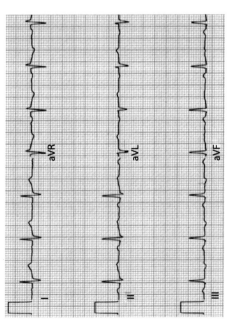

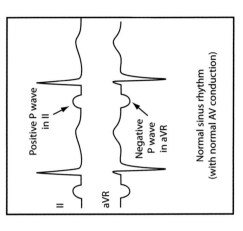

Positive P wave in II

Negative P wave in aVR

Normal sinus rhythm (with normal AV conduction)

Figure 9.2:

We often shorten "normal sinus rhythm with normal AV conduction" to "normal sinus rhythm." Obviously the sinus node could still be generating depolarization but if atrioventricular conduction was blocked every P wave would not be associated with a QRS (this cause of bradycardia is covered in Chapter 10). So we should always remember that when we say a patient has "normal sinus rhythm," we are really saying two things: the sinus node is generating the beat and atrioventricular conduction is normal. In this example the P waves are negative in aVR and positive in lead II. The PR interval is 0.20 s, which is the upper limit of normal. It is hoped that after reading the first portion of the book you would have noted the inverted T wave in lead III that could still be a normal finding since there are no accompanying T wave changes or QRS abnormalities in the other inferior leads.

Regular Rhythm

Normal Sinus Rhythm (artifact)

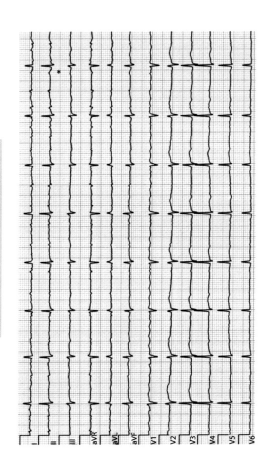

Figure 9.3:

Sometimes electrical signals from other electrical equipment will interfere with the ECG recording. In this case low amplitude from an implanted muscle stimulator is interfering with the ECG but a P wave can be observed (*). This patient has a normal heart rhythm.

Regular Rhythm

Ectopic atrial rhythm

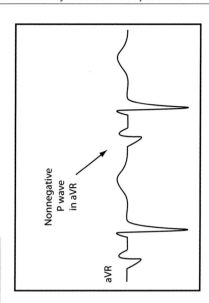

Nonnegative
P wave
in aVR

aVR

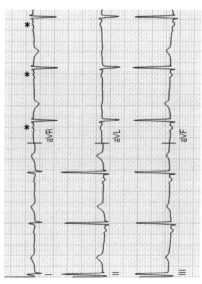

Figure 9.4:

In an ectopic atrial rhythm, a site other than the sinus node depolarizes the atrium. In ectopic atrial rhythm the P wave will not be positive in lead II and negative in aVR*. The shape of the P wave will be dependent on the site of the ectopic atrial focus. In this example the ectopic atrial rhythm is being generated from a site in the lower part of the atria since the P waves are negative in the inferior leads (atrial depolarization must be travelling away from these leads). Since the P wave is positive in aVL and flat or partially negative in aVR, the ectopic site is also probably within the right atrium. Generally ectopic atrial rhythm is of no clinical consequence.

Regular Rhythm

Junctional Rhythm

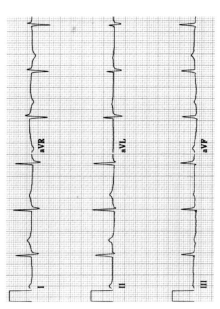

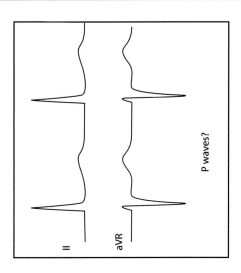

P waves?

Figure 9.5:
Generally, the sinus node has the fastest pacemaker rate of all of the cardiac tissues and "drives" cardiac activity. However, in some cases the AV nodal area can depolarize faster than the sinus node and a junctional rhythm will be observed. In junctional rhythm, since the AV node is generating the heart beat, there is no P wave before the QRS complex. Junctional rhythm generally has no clinical consequence but a slow junctional rhythm (Chapter 10 on bradycardia) may be a sign of sinus node dysfunction.

Regular rhythm

Sinus rhythm with first degree AV block

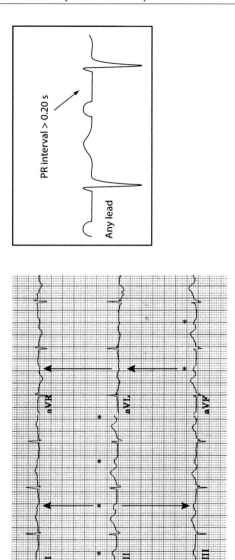

Figure 9.6:

In this example, the inverted P wave in aVR and positive P wave in II is evidence that the sinus node is responsible for atrial depolarization (*). However, the PR interval is abnormally prolonged (0.36 s). Any PR interval > 0.20 s is classified as first degree AV block. In this case there is "normal" sinus rhythm (the P waves are being generated at a normal rate) but atrioventricular conduction is not "normal." Oftentimes, new ECG readers look for a P wave in front of every QRS as their definition of "normal sinus rhythm." As illustrated in this example, evaluating the relationship between P waves and QRS complexes is a measure of AV node and His Purkinje function. Finally, this ECG illustrates an important advantage to digital ECG recording in which signals are acquired simultaneously. If a P wave is easily identified in one lead (II and aVF), the leads above and below can be evaluated and more subtle deflections that represent P waves can be identified (arrows).

Irregular Rhythm

Sinus arrhythmia

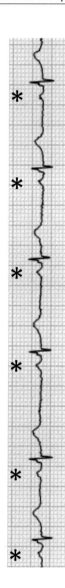

Figure 9.7:

The most common cause of an irregular heart rate in young adults is normal irregular depolarization of the sinus node. The rate of sinus node depolarization changes as metabolic need changes. When we exercise the sinus rate increases because of more sympathetic nerve (the "adrenalin" system) activity. In young people the sinus rate will change fairly dramatically simply with normal breathing. In sinus arrhythmia all of the P waves (*) have the same shape but the interval between P waves varies.

Irregular Rhythm

Premature atrial contractions

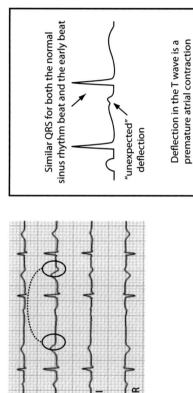

Similar QRS for both the normal sinus rhythm beat and the early beat

"unexpected" deflection

Deflection in the T wave is a premature atrial contraction

I

II

III

aVR

Figure 9.8:

Another common cause of an irregular heartbeat is a premature atrial contraction. Another site within the atria, other than the sinus node, depolarizes early. This leads to an early P wave that often can be found in the preceding T wave (circled areas). Since the ventricles are still activated normally by the His Purkinje system the QRS complex comes early but has a normal shape similar to the QRS complexes produced by the sinus beats. Premature atrial contractions generally have no clinical consequence but in some people can initiate atrial fibrillation (Chapter 11, Figure 11.4).

Irregular Rhythm

Premature junctional contractions

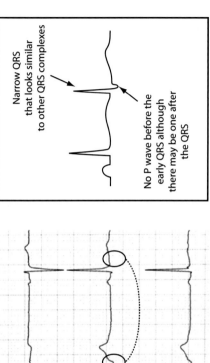

Narrow QRS
that looks similar
to other QRS complexes

No P wave before the
early QRS although
there may be one after
the QRS

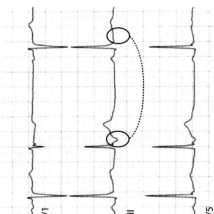

V1

II

V5

Figure 9.9:

Another cause of an early beat is premature depolarization from the AV nodal area. In this case the early QRS complex will be the same as the sinus rhythm QRS complexes but there will be no early P wave before the early QRS complex. Sometimes the premature junctional beat will lead to both ventricular contraction and atrial contraction. In this case the atria are depolarized abnormally from "low to high" so the P wave is inverted. This backwards depolarization is usually called retrograde conduction. If retrograde conduction is very fast the P wave might be observed just before the QRS complex (extremely rare), if retrograde conduction and ventricular depolarization are similar the smaller P wave will

be obscured by the QRS complex (most common), and if retrograde conduction is slower than ventricular depolarization the inverted P wave will be seen in the ST segment. Again, comparing the QRS, ST segment and T wave for both the normal beat and the early beat is extremely useful. In this case the early beat has a negative deflection in the ST segment that is not seen in the normal beat (circles). This "unexpected" deflection must be a P wave and confirms that the early beat arose from the AV node. Premature junctional complexes have very little clinical consequence other than being an ECG oddity.

Irregular Rhythm

Premature ventricular contractions

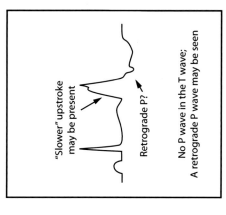

"Slower" upstroke may be present

Retrograde P?

No P wave in the T wave; A retrograde P wave may be seen

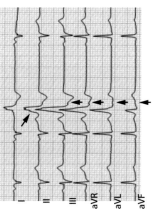

I

II

III

aVR

aVL

aVF

Figure 9.10:

Sometimes early activity arises from ventricular tissue to produce a premature ventricular complex. Since premature ventricular complexes do not use the normal His Purkinje system for ventricular depolarization, the QRS complex is wide and bizarre, appearing often with an initial upstroke or downstroke that is less steep (arrow). Retrograde atrial contraction can sometimes be seen after the QRS complex (vertical arrows) but may be very subtle. Premature

ventricular contractions may be a marker for increased risk of ventricular arrhythmias but may also be benign and of no clinical consequence. A general rule (a "glass bead" rather than a pearl) is that premature ventricular contractions are "bad" if they are associated with the presence of other structural heart disease (reduced heart function, etc.) and "Not much to worry about" if the patient has no other heart abnormalities.

Irregular Rhythm

Premature atrial contractions (with aberrant conduction)

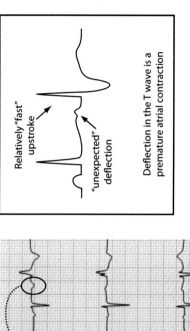

Relatively "fast" upstroke

"unexpected" deflection

Deflection in the T wave is a premature atrial contraction

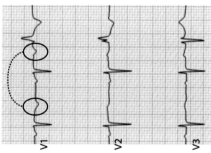

V1

V2

V3

Figure 9.11:

Not all early QRS wide QRS complexes are from premature ventricular contractions. Another cause of an early wide QRS complex is a premature atrial contraction that is associated with aberrant or abnormal conduction. In this case, as the depolarization from the premature atrial contraction reaches the His Purkinje system, one of the bundle branches (usually the right bundle branch) is refractory (cannot conduct) and the wave of depolarization only travels down one of the bundles. Bundle branch block leads to sequential activation of the ventricles and a wide QRS complex. Identification of a premature atrial contraction with aberrant conduction requires identification of the early atrial depolarization. As reviewed in Figure 9.8, careful comparison of the T waves for the beat before the early beat and a later regular beat will help (circles).

Irregular Rhythm

Competing pacemakers

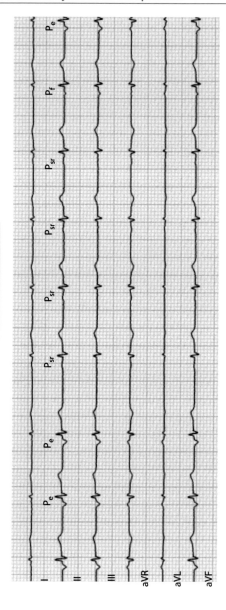

Figure 9.12:

Sometimes irregular heart rhythms can be seen when different sites within the atria have similar rates or irregular and "compete." In this example, a site from the lower atrium is faster than the sinus node and produces a P wave that is inverted in the inferior leads (P_e) and an ectopic atrial rhythm. When this "pacemaker" pauses, the sinus node takes over and produces a normal upright P wave (P_{sr}) and a short run of sinus rhythm. However, the lower atrial site begins to depolarize again at a rate faster than the sinus node and gradually takes over. Notice that there is one P wave (P_f) that is a "fusion" beat where atrial depolarization is due to both the ectopic site and the sinus node and the P wave has an intermediate morphology between the P wave from the ectopic atrial rhythm and the P wave produced by the sinus node.

Irregular Rhythm

Atrial fibrillation

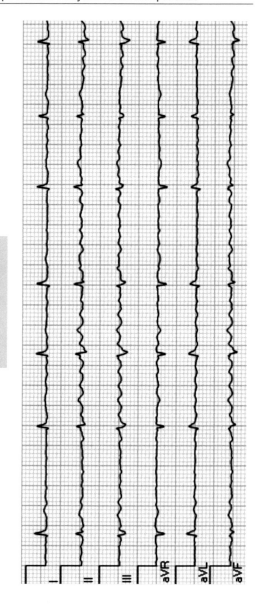

Figure 9.13:

Another cause of an irregular rhythm with a relatively normal heart rate is atrial fibrillation. In atrial fibrillation, the atria are activated continuously by multiple atrial waves of depolarization. Atrial fibrillation is generally associated with a rapid ventricular rate because rapid atrial activation leads to rapid ventricular rates but in some cases, if the AV node does not conduct rapidly, atrial fibrillation can be associated with relatively normal rates although the rhythm will be irregular. Atrial fibrillation is covered extensively in Chapter 11, Figures 11.3, 11.4, and 11.7 and of all the arrhythmias it is the most prevalent and associated with the most hospital admissions.

CHAPTER 10

Arrhythmias: Bradycardia

There are only two general causes of slow heart rates: Failure of the sinus node to deliver normal impulses or depolarization is blocked between the atrium and the ventricles (atrioventricular or AV block) (Figure 10.1). Although someone new to clinical medicine might say, "who cares? A slow heart rate is a slow heart rate," it is very important to make this distinction as the management can vary dramatically. The ECG can provide definitive information on the specific site of the problem.

In sinus node dysfunction, since the sinus node does not generate an impulse at the normal rate there are fewer P waves than expected. There are many manifestations of sinus node dysfunction including sinus pauses, sinus bradycardia, ectopic atrial rhythm, or junctional rhythm. In ectopic atrial rhythm and junctional rhythm, the sinus rate is so slow that a subsidiary pacemaker, either from another region in the atrium or the AV node, must take over and "drive" the heart. We introduced ectopic atria rhythms and junctional rhythms in the last chapter. Ectopic atrial rhythms and junctional rhythms can be observed if these sites have more rapid activity than the sinus node or in the case of sinus node dysfunction if the sinus node pacemaker activity slows. These two situations can generally be differentiated by rate, the arbitrary cut-off for an abnormal sinus rate is 50 beats per minute and the AV junction has a spontaneous rate of about 35–50 beats per minute. If junctional rhythm is observed because of more rapid junctional activity the heart rate will be > 50 beats per minute and if junctional rhythm is observed because of sinus node dysfunction, the heart rate will be < 50 beats per minute.

In AV block the site of block is usually in the AV node or in the His bundle since these two structures, in most cases, form the only axis for AV conduction. Clinically AV block is classified by the relationship between the P waves and the QRS complexes. In first degree AV block

ECG Interpretation for Everyone: An On-The-Spot Guide, First Edition.
Fred Kusumoto and Pam Bernath.
© 2012 John Wiley & Sons, Ltd. Published 2012 by John Wiley & Sons, Ltd.

(introduced in Chapter 9, Figure 9.6) there is a one to one relationship between the P waves and the QRS complexes but the time required for AV conduction is prolonged (> 0.20 s). First degree AV block does not cause slow heart rates in and of itself since every P wave is conducted to the ventricles. In second degree AV block some but not all P waves are conducted to the ventricles and in third degree heart block there is no relationship between P waves and QRS complexes. It is important to remember that AV block is a normal response in the setting of rapid atrial activity. For example, if the atria were to suddenly start to beat at 300 times a minute (as in atrial flutter, Chapter 11, Figure 11.6), the AV node acts to limit the number of impulses that propagate to the ventricles and prevents rapid ventricular rates. Think of the AV node as a regulator that "protects" the ventricle from atrial arrhythmias. The corollary of this point is that abnormal AV conduction should only be identified if the P waves have a normal rate.

Second degree AV block is further classified into different types depending on the exact relationship between P waves and QRS complexes. In 1924, Woldemar Mobitz classified 2° AV blocks into Type I or Type II. In Type I block there is gradual prolongation of the PR interval until a QRS complex is dropped. Type I block is most commonly called Wenckebach block in honor of Karl Wenckebach who first described this unusual conduction pattern in the late 1800s by carefully evaluating the relationship between the venous and arterial pulsations without the aid of the ECG (pretty impressive). In Type II block the PR interval remains constant and there is a sudden dropped QRS complex. The distinction between Type I and Type II block is very easy to make from the ECG. Simply measure the PR interval before and after the P wave associated with the dropped QRS complex. If the PR intervals are different Type I block is present and if they are the same Type II block is present. The distinction between Type I and Type II block is extremely important. In Type I block, the site of block is usually within the AV node so that if complete AV block develops the patient is usually left with a junctional rhythm with a heart rate of 35–50 bpm. The presence of Type II block suggests that the site of block is "below the AV node" within the His bundle (infranodal block). In this case, if complete AV block develops the patient is dependent on a pacemaker within ventricular tissues for the generation of QRS complexes. These ventricular sites are associated with very slow heart rates and are extremely unreliable and can stop suddenly.

Sinus rhythm

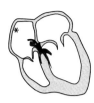
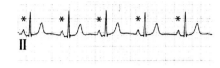

Sinus node dysfunction with junctional escape rhythm

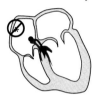
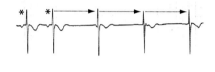

AV block with junctional escape rhythm

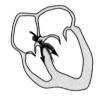
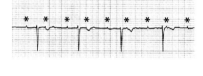

Figure 10.1:

Bradycardia can develop from either failure of the sinus node to initiate depolarization (sinus node dysfunction) or once the atrium is depolarized, atrioventricular block. The two forms of bradycardia can easily be differentiated by the ECG: in sinus node dysfunction not enough P waves are generated, while in AV block there are "enough" P waves, but they do not conduct to the ventricles in a normal fashion. In the example, since the sinus node is not depolarizing normally, a subsidiary site, the AV node, "takes over" depolarizing the heart. Junctional beats in this case can be identified because the QRS complex is not preceded by a P wave. In the example of AV block, there is no AV conduction, so the AV node region also generates the QRS complexes but

There are two situations that do not "fit" into the Type I and Type II classification system for AV block. In the first, every other P wave is associated with a QRS complex. In 2:1 AV block although the PR intervals are the same before and after the blocked P wave, 2:1 AV block can be due to block within the AV node or infranodal. In most cases of 2:1 block the patient will have a few consecutive P waves that conduct to the ventricles so that the distinction between Type I and Type II can be made. Generally since Type I AV block is much more common than Type II block, intermittent periods with gradual prolongation of the PR interval will be observed between periods of 2:1 AV block. In the second situation called advanced AV block, two or more consecutive nonconducted P waves are present. In this case three or more P waves are presented between QRS complexes but some P waves conduct so that some AV conduction is present.

Although discussed earlier, there are two common circumstances where AV conduction is normal but are classified incorrectly as 2° degree AV block. In the first a premature atrial contraction (PAC) is not associated with a QRS complex (often called a "blocked PAC" in clinical shorthand). The second situation is an abnormal atrial rate associated with block in AV conduction. The AV node has decremental conduction properties so both of these responses are actually normal. In order to make the diagnosis of AV block, the P waves must be regular and with a normal rate.

In complete heart block (3° AV block) there is no relationship between P waves and QRS complexes. If the block is within the AV node a regular narrow QRS rhythm or junctional rhythm will be observed. This can be a source of confusion since junctional rhythm is also a manifestation of sinus node dysfunction. The difference is that in complete heart block P waves are present and do not conduct to the ventricles and in junctional rhythm due to sinus node dysfunction P waves generated by the sinus node will not be seen. If complete heart block due to infranodal block develops, the escape QRS complex will be wide.

Figure 10.1: (*Cont'd*)
unlike sinus node dysfunction P waves at a normal rate are present. (With permission, taken from FM Kusumoto, *ECG Interpretation:* *From Pathophysiology to Clinical Application*, Springer, New York, NY, 2009.)

The distinction between 2° degree AV block and complete heart block seems confusing at first glance. For example, how do I differentiate between advanced AV block and complete heart block? Actually there is a practical way for the ECG to help. In 2° AV block, generally the QRS rhythm is irregular because of some conducted P waves while in complete AV block the QRS rhythm will be regular. This practical method helps in another situation. In atrial fibrillation, the atria are activated irregularly and in turn this leads to an irregular QRS rhythm. In patients with atrial fibrillation and complete AV block, a *regular* slow QRS rhythm will be observed.

Sinus Node dysfunction (Not enough P waves)

Artifact

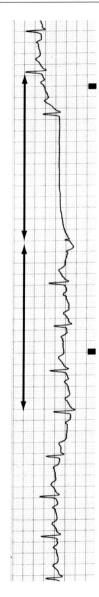

Figure 10.2:

Particularly with rhythm strips, artifact (in reference to the ECG, artifact refers to any condition in which an external source or problem causes a change in the ECG recording rather than an actual signal generated by cardiac activity) can lead to apparent asystole. The most common cause of this problem is that one of the leads temporarily loses skin contact. In this case, artifact is confirmed since the sinus rate is unchanged before and after the apparent pause (the R-R intervals denoted by the double-headed arrows are constant) and a small "partial" signal also be identified. Obviously it is important to determine whether the patient has symptoms during any "arrhythmia" episode. Although absence of symptoms does not "rule out" arrhythmias, in almost all diseases the presence of symptoms is associated with a worse prognosis.

Sinus Node dysfunction (Not enough P waves)

Sinus pause with idioventricular rhythm

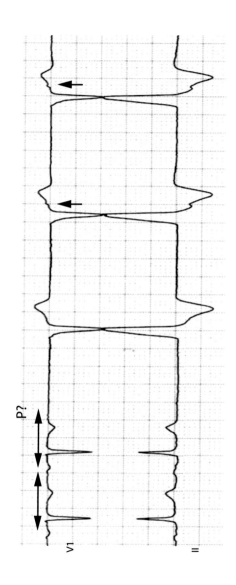

Figure 10.3:

In this case of sinus node dysfunction, the sinus node stops depolarizing so no P waves are observed but the resulting QRS is wide and very slow because the subsidiary AV node pacemaker also did not depolarize normally. Ventricular pacemakers such as in this case are slower and notoriously unreliable (they can stop suddenly) and patients are at higher risk for developing significant symptoms. Compare this to the middle panel of Figure 10.1. In

Figure 10.1, when a sinus pause occurs the AV node "takes over." In this case, a deflection after the QRS complex due to retrograde depolarization of the atria can be observed (arrows). The AV node is a "two-way street" and can conduct both forward and backward. Normally since the sinus node has the fastest pacemaker activity, only forward conduction through the AV node and His bundle is observed.

Sinus Node dysfunction (Not enough P waves)

Sinus node exit block

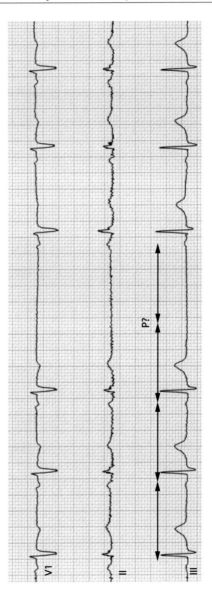

Figure 10.4:

There are many forms of sinus node dysfunction. In this case, instead of a prolonged pause, a single P wave is dropped. This condition is sometimes called sinus node exit block because it is thought to be due to block of depolarization from the sinus node to surrounding atrial tissue.

Atrioventricular block (Ps without QRSs)

Wenckebach 2° AV block (Mobitz Type I)

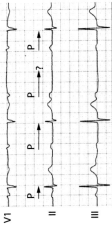

Figure 10.5:

There are several patterns of 2° AV block that have been identified by ECG. In all forms of 2° AV block some but not all P waves conduct to the ventricles to produce a QRS complex. Originally Mobitz described two forms: Type I and Type II. This is an example of Type I AV block (more commonly called Wenckebach block) that is characterized by progressive prolongation of the PR interval (arrows) until finally there is a dropped QRS (?) due to AV block of atrial depolarization. In any case of AV block it is important to make a clinical guess at the site of block. Block within the AV node while abnormal carries a better prognosis than block within the His bundle. Almost all cases of Mobitz Type I block associated with a narrow QRS complex are due to block in the AV node.

Atrioventricular block (Ps without QRSs)

Wenckebach 2° AV block
(with right bundle branch block)

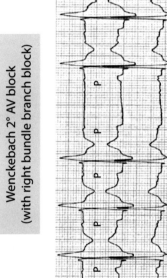

Figure 10.6:

This is another example of Mobitz Type I block identified by progressive PR interval prolongation before the dropped QRS complex. In this case, the QRS is wide due to right bundle branch block (Chapter7, Figure 7.5). Generally any time Mobitz Type I block is identified, the site of block is in the AV node, although in this case the presence of accompanying right bundle branch block is evidence that some His Purkinje disease is present.

Atrioventricular block (Ps without QRSs)

Mobitz Type II 2° AV block

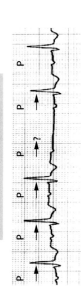

Figure 10.7:

In Mobitz Type II block, the PR interval remains constant before a P wave is associated with a dropped QRS complex (?). Mobitz Type II block is important to identify because it is generally due to block in the His bundle region and carries a worse prognosis than block in the AV node (mainly due to the slower and more unreliable ventricular pacemakers that would have to depolarize the heart if complete heart block were to develop). Although most textbooks emphasize evaluating successive PR intervals prior to the P wave with the dropped QRS, it is often easier to simply evaluate the PR interval before and after the P wave without the QRS complex. If the PR intervals are different, Type I block is present, and if the PR intervals are the same, the patient has Type II block.

"Atrioventricular block"
(Ps without QRSs)

Blocked premature atrial contractions

Figure 10.8:

It is important to remember that abnormal AV block can generally be identified only when the P wave rate is constant. In this case there are premature atrial contractions (PAC) that do not result in ventricular conduction and a QRS complex because the AV node is refractory. This condition is sometimes misidentified as abnormal AV block. Remember from Chapter 3 that AV nodal conduction delay is important to allow efficient filling of the ventricles from atrial contraction. In addition, as we will learn in Chapter 11, by acting as a "limiter" the AV node prevents rapid atrial activity from resulting in rapid ventricular conduction.

Atrioventricular block
(P's without QRS's)

2:1 2° AV block

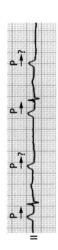

Figure 10.9:

This is an example of 2:1 AV block. The P wave rate is regular but every other P wave does not conduct to the ventricles and leads to an absent QRS complex (?). When 2:1 AV block is present it is impossible to classify the AV block as Type I or Type II although generally there will be periods where two consecutive P waves conduct to the ventricle and the PR interval can be examined for any changes and the PR interval before and after the P wave with the dropped QRS complex can be evaluated.

Atrioventricular block
(Ps without QRSs)

Advanced 2° AV block

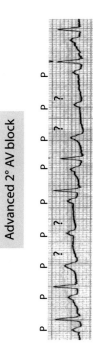

Figure 10.10:
In advanced AV block, some conduction from the atrium to the ventricles occurs but several consecutive P waves do not conduct to the ventricles (?). While there is some AV communication, the presence of consecutive P waves at normal rates that do not conduct provides strong evidence that AV conduction is tenuous at best.

Atrioventricular block (P's without QRS's)

Complete heart block (3° AV block)

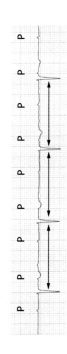

Figure 10.11:

In complete heart block, there is no AV conduction and the patient is dependent on an intrinsic pacemaker below the site of block for ventricular depolarization. Complete heart block will be associated with a regular slow rate because no

P waves lead to ventricular depolarization (double-headed arrows). In contrast, in almost all cases of 2° AV block, the rhythm will be irregular due to variable AV conduction.

Atrioventricular block ("Ps" without QRSs)

Complete heart block (3° AV block) in atrial fibrillation

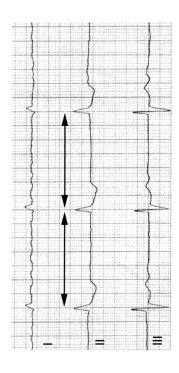

Figure 10.12:

In atrial fibrillation, the atria are activated rapidly and chaotically usually leading to rapid and irregular heart rates (Chapter 11, Figure 11.3). In the setting of complete heart block, the ventricular rate will be regular (double-headed arrows) despite the presence of atrial fibrillation. In the past this was almost always due to digoxin toxicity.

Atrioventricular block
(Ps without QRSs)

Severe advanced AV block (2° AV block)

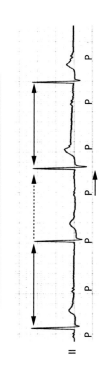

Figure 10.13:

Using the strict definition of complete heart block (no AV conduction), the QRS complexes will generally be regular. In this example, the fourth P wave conducts leading to one slightly early QRS complex (third QRS). The first, second, and fourth QRS complexes arise from the junction since they have a regular slow rate (double-headed arrows). Although this is not a case of complete heart block, clinically this condition would be treated in exactly the same way as complete heart block.

Atrioventricular block (Ps without QRSs)

Advanced 2° AV block (with bundle branch block)

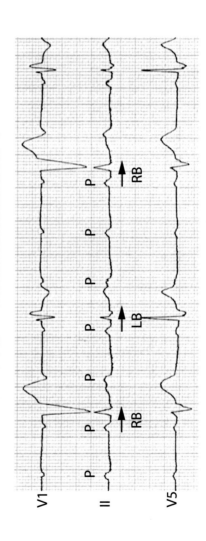

Figure 10.14:

In the setting of AV block, it is important to evaluate the QRS complexes-both from lower subsidiary pacemakers and for conducted beats. This information is critical for evaluating short-term and long-term prognosis. In this case of advanced 2° AV block (consecutive nonconducted P waves), when atrioventricular conduction does occur sometimes only the right bundle (RB) conducts producing a QRS with a left bundle branch block morphology (wide negative QS complex) and at other times only the left bundle (LB) conducts producing a QRS with a right bundle branch block morphology. This condition is particularly worrisome and the clinician should be very concerned about the development of P waves without QRS complexes (no heart rate = a bad thing).

CHAPTER 11

Arrhythmias: Tachycardia

Okay, take a very deep breath as this chapter is by far and away the most difficult to get through (hopefully you are not already grumbling "Oh dear, the first ten were awfully tough"). At first glance, the material appears very dense with a lot of information. Sadly you might be right about the quantity of material, but it is hoped this chapter will provide an outline to make the material easier to organize. However, the ECG is the fundamental diagnostic tool for evaluating rapid heart rates. In fact, if at all possible (sometimes the clinician is limited because of hemodynamic collapse), any patient who is thought to have an abnormal rapid heart rate should receive a 12 lead ECG as soon as possible. Once mastered, the ability to quickly evaluate an ECG is an essential skill necessary for taking care of critically ill patients.

From an anatomic standpoint, rapid heart rates can be due to abnormally rapid activity from three sites: the atria, AV junction, or the ventricles. The fourth cause of tachycardia uses an abnormal muscular connection between the atria and ventricles (accessory pathway) that is used as the essential component in the tachycardia (Figure 11.1).

Although this anatomic classification is extremely helpful for remembering the different types of tachycardia and will be used for the remainder of the chapter, clinically the ECG is used to make a distinction between narrow complex tachycardias and wide complex tachycardias. In narrow complex tachycardia, the QRS has a normal appearance with an rS complex in V_1 and a width < 0.12 s. The normal QRS complex means that the ventricles are being activated normally using the His Purkinje tissue and generally rules out a tachycardia arising solely from ventricular tissue (ventricular tachycardia). In wide complex tachycardias, the focus will be on deciding whether the patient has ventricular

ECG Interpretation for Everyone: An On-The-Spot Guide, First Edition.
Fred Kusumoto and Pam Bernath.
© 2012 John Wiley & Sons, Ltd. Published 2012 by John Wiley & Sons, Ltd.

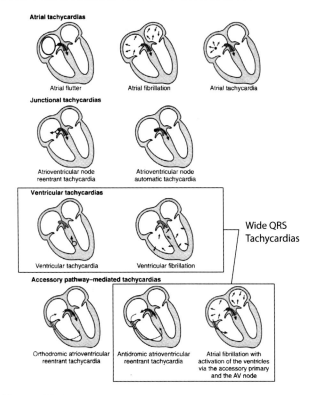

Figure 11.1:

Anatomic types of tachycardia. The ventricular tachycardias and the accessory pathway mediated tachycardias in which the ventricles are activated by the accessory pathway always are associated with a wide complex tachycardia (Wide QRS tachycardia). The other tachycardias are usually associated with a narrow QRS tachycardia and are grouped together as supraventricular tachycardias. Any supraventricular tachycardia can be associated with aberrant conduction and produce a wide complex tachycardia. (Adapted with permission from FM Kusumoto, *Cardiovascular Pathophysiology*, Hayes Barton Press, Raleigh, NC, 2004.)

tachycardia or one of the supraventricular tachycardias with abnormal or aberrant conduction. Ventricular tachycardia is generally more likely to be life-threatening, while the supraventricular tachycardia, although it may be associated with significant symptoms, is generally better tolerated. The presence of a narrow QRS on the ECG is a first form of "triage," and essentially rules out ventricular tachycardia.

Narrow QRS tachycardias are generally grouped together and called supraventricular tachycardias, to emphasize that ventricular tachycardia is not present. If we return to our anatomic classification scheme, supraventricular tachycardia can have three anatomic causes: atrial tachycardias, junctional tachycardias, or accessory pathway mediated tachycardias. In atrial tachycardia, the cause of tachycardia is solely within atrial tissue. This could be a site or sites within the atria that are depolarizing (or "firing") abnormally fast or a reentrant circuit within the atria.

We now have to take a slight "detour" and talk about the difference between automaticity and reentry (Figure 11.2). Automaticity is very easy to understand conceptually as a single or several rapidly blinking lights that cause rapid atrial activity. On the other hand, reentry is not very intuitive and can be one of the most confusing subjects for students learning about arrhythmias. However, a cursory understanding of reentry is necessary for analyzing the ECG. In reentry a "substrate" consisting of two parallel pathways with connected ends and different electrical properties is present. Generally, a wave of activation travels through both sides of the pathway equally. But a premature stimulation can lead to conduction down only one pathway, due to block in the other pathway. In some cases, the impulse can turn around and travel backwards up the parallel pathway, setting up a continual loop of depolarization. The analogy that is often used is a dog chasing its tail. The electrical activity continues to circle on the two pathways until one of the arms blocks suddenly and the tachycardia stops. Tachycardias due to reentry tend to start suddenly and stop abruptly. Although it might not first seem obvious, parallel electrical pathways are quite common in the diseased heart due to the development of scar tissue and natural barriers, e.g. the entrance of the *vena cavae* into the right atrium (see the discussion on atrial flutter which follows).

So now back to our discussion of atrial tachycardias. An atrial tachycardia due to a single rapidly depolarizing site is formally called a focal atrial tachycardia, although to add to the confusion these arrhythmias are often just called atrial tachycardias. If three or more sites are depolarizing

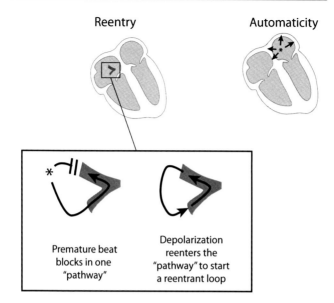

Figure 11.2:

The two cellular/tissue causes of tachycardia are automaticity and reentry. In automaticity a site or sites within the heart begins to depolarize abnormally fast. In this example an automatic site is located within the atria. In reentry, a "substrate" of two parallel "pathways" is present. The pathways can be anywhere and are separated by fibrosis or a normal anatomic structure (e.g. the inferior vena cava). In this example the two "pathways" are shown in the right atrium. A premature beat blocks in one "pathway" and conducts in only one "pathway." The wave of depolarization turns around by depolarizing the other "pathway" and a reentrant circuit develops. Reentry requires both "substrate"-two pathways with different electrical properties and a "trigger" to initiate the reentry.

abnormally, the arrhythmia is called a multifocal atrial tachycardia. An atrial tachycardia due to reentry within atrial tissue is called atrial flutter (Figure 11.1).

Tachycardias that arise from junctional tissue are usually due to small reentrant circuits that are confined to the AV node and adjacent atrial tissue (AV node reentrant tachycardia or AVNRT). In rare cases (usually children), an unusual arrhythmia called junctional ectopic tachycardia (JET) due to an automatic focus from junctional tissue can be observed (Figure 11.1).

The final distinct anatomic cause of supraventricular tachycardia uses an accessory pathway. Usually the AV node is the only electrical connection between the atria and the ventricles, but in some cases a strand of tissue that forms an additional electrical connection between the atria and ventricles called an accessory pathway is present (Chapter 7, Figures 7.9 and 7.10 and Chapter 8, Figure 8.3). The coexistence of the AV node and an accessory pathway are the perfect conditions for the development of reentry. Under normal conditions, atrial depolarization travels down both the accessory pathway and the AV node to depolarize the ventricles. A premature atrial contraction can sometimes block in the accessory pathway and conduct solely down the AV node to activate the ventricles. Ventricular depolarization may activate the ventricular end of the accessory pathway and the depolarization can travel "backwards" up the accessory pathway to depolarize the atria and initiate a reentrant circuit (the dog chasing its tail). This type of tachycardia is called atrioventricular reentrant tachycardia or AVRT and leads to a rapid supraventricular tachycardia since the ventricles are being depolarized normally via the AV node and His Purkinje system.

Although there are obvious complexities and subtleties, in general, when evaluating a supraventricular tachycardia there are two considerations: determining whether the rhythm is regular or irregular and identifying atrial activity.

Irregular supraventricular tachycardias are generally due to tachycardias from rapid atrial activity (atrial tachycardias) (Table 11.1). Rapid atrial activity can have several forms. The most common cause of an irregular supraventricular tachycardia is atrial fibribrillation where irregular, continuous, and chaotic atrial activity called fibrillatory waves is observed. In atrial fibrillation, the pulse and ventricular rhythm is extremely irregular because of irregular activation of the ventricles via the AV node. Several other forms of rapid atrial activity can also cause irregular rhythms. In multifocal atrial tachycardia, several different sites within the atria alternatively activate the atria. Think of rapidly blinking lights from different sites and rates within the atria. Both atrial fibrillation and multifocal atrial tachycardia cause irregular rapid heart rhythms, and the distinction between the two is made by the ECG. In multifocal atrial tachycardia, the

Table 11.1: Causes of supraventricular tachycardia

ECG Rhythm	Possibilities
Irregular	Atrial tachycardias
	• Atrial fibrillation
	• Multifocal atrial tachycardia
	• Atrial flutter/focal atrial tachycardia with variable AV conduction
Regular	Atrial flutter/focal atrial tachycardia
	Junctional tachycardia
	Accessory Pathway-mediated (AVRT,ORT)

atria are depolarized as a single wave, albeit at abnormal rates and from different sites, so discrete P waves of different shapes are observed. In atrial fibrillation, the atria are not depolarized as single waves of activity and rather by continuous ever-changing smaller waves of activity. One way to think about the differences between multifocal atrial tachycardia and atrial fibrillation is the motion of water at the beach or in a rapidly flowing river. At the beach, waves break at irregular intervals but between the waves there is no activity. In contrast, in a rapidly flowing river, multiple different waves are continuously slowing in an ever-changing pattern with no quiescent period.

Usually focal atrial tachycardias and atrial flutters lead to regular rapid rhythms but in some cases regular rapid atrial activity can lead to some irregularity of the QRS complexes due to variable conduction. However, even in this case there will be periods of regular tachycardia, and when an irregular tachycardia develops fixed intervals will still be observed since the atria are being depolarized regularly. This pattern is often called "regularly irregular" to differentiate it from atrial fibrillation and multifocal atrial tachycardia which are associated with very irregular QRS rhythms because the atria are being activated irregularly (often referred to as "irregularly irregular"). In some cases of atrial fibrillation, large areas of tissue are activated relatively regularly, leading to the appearance of larger "flutter" waves, particularly in lead V_1, and this is sometimes called "coarse" atrial fibrillation. The distinction between atrial flutter and atrial fibrillation is usually made by the QRS rhythm; if the QRS rhythm is irregularly irregular, it is classified as atrial fibrillation, and if there is some pattern of regularity, it is called atrial flutter or atrial tachycardia.

A regular supraventricular tachycardia can be caused by a regular atrial tachycardia or atrial flutter, a rhythm arising from the AV junction, and finally in one of the tachycardias that use an accessory pathway. Atrial tachycardia and atrial flutter have already been described and if AV conduction is constant, a regular tachycardia is observed. In most cases every other depolarization of atrium conducts to the ventricle (2:1 conduction). For example, the most common form of atrial flutter depolarizes the atrium at a regular rate of 300 beats per minute, if every other depolarization is conducted to the ventricles, the resulting ventricular rate will be 150 beats per minute. Fast but probably a lot more stable than a heart rate of 300 bpm! Careful inspection of the ECG is required to identify the P waves.

Tachycardias arising from the AV junction area are usually due to a small reentrant circuit due to small parallel inputs into or within the AV node. Since the junction is driving the heart, the ventricles are activated via the His Purkinje system and the atria are activated "backwards" from the AV node region. Since the atria and ventricles are activated simultaneously the P wave is sometimes obscured by the QRS complex or seen at the end of the QRS complex.

As discussed previously in this chapter, patients with an accessory pathway can develop supraventricular tachycardia. In contrast to tachycardias arising from the junction the ventricles and atria are activated sequentially one after the other. For this reason, the P waves are typically observed after the QRS complex within the ST segment. As will be emphasized in the figures, identification of the P waves can provide important clues for determining what type of tachycardia is present.

One last confusing point about supraventricular tachycardias is the "alphabet soup" of abbreviations used to describe them:

SVT: Supraventricular tachycardia – a generic term used to describe any fast heart rhythm with a normal QRS complex.

PSVT: Paroxysmal supraventricular tachycardia – an SVT that occurs sporadically and starts suddenly and stops suddenly.

AVNRT: AV node reentrant tachycardia – a reentrant tachycardia with all of the components for the reentrant circuit within the AV node and /or adjacent tissue.

AVRT: Atrioventricular reentrant tachycardia –a reentrant tachycardia that uses an accessory pathway and the AV node as two "limbs" of a reentrant circuit.

ORT: Orthodromic reciprocating tachycardia – the specific form of AVRT in which the AV node activates the ventricles and the accessory pathway activates the atria. The term "ortho" comes from the Greek word "normal or standard" and "dromic" for direction to describe the normal direction of AV conduction in this type of tachycardia that results in a narrow complex tachycardia.

A wide QRS tachycardia is also called wide complex tachycardia. In this case, the ventricles are not being activated normally by the His Purkinje system. Any of the supraventricular tachycardias can cause a wide QRS tachycardia if there is abnormal or aberrant conduction in the His Purkinje system, often collectively referred to as "SVT with aberrancy." But wide QRS tachycardia can also be caused by rapid ventricular activation due to automaticity or a reentrant circuit within ventricular tissue. Any tachycardia that is due solely to abnormal activation of ventricular tissue is called ventricular tachycardia. Although both SVT with aberrancy and ventricular tachycardia can be associated with significant symptoms, rapid identification of ventricular tachycardia is critical since ventricular tachycardia is often unstable and can lead to sudden death. For this reason, the ECG is very useful for first identifying whether a tachycardia is wide complex or narrow complex (SVT) and second, for differentiating between ventricular tachycardia and SVT with aberrancy. The ECG clues for identifying ventricular tachycardia are provided in Figures 11.17 through 11.24.

Irregular Narrow QRS tachycardia

Atrial fibrillation

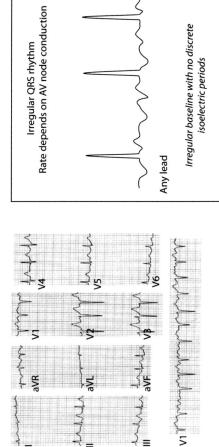

Irregular QRS rhythm
Rate depends on AV node conduction

Any lead

Irregular baseline with no discrete isoelectric periods

Figure 11.3:

Background: Atrial fibrillation is the most common arrhythmia in medicine. In atrial fibrillation there are several simultaneous waves of atrial depolarization that change and depolarize the atria in a random fashion.

ECG: The ECG in atrial fibrillation shows chaotic atrial activity with no "quiescent" period at baseline because of continuous depolarization of the atria. The ventricles depolarize irregularly due to irregular activation of the AV node and His Purkinje system. The ventricular rate in atrial fibrillation depends on AV node function. If the AV node is diseased or abnormal due to drug, the ventricular rate in atrial fibrillation will be normal or even slow (Chapter 9, Figure 9.13 and Chapter 10, Figure 10.12).

Clinical Issues: Atrial fibrillation can lead to significant tiredness and fatigue due to the rapid ventricular rate and loss of atrial contribution to ventricular filling. However, in some cases patients are only minimally symptomatic and in some cases completely asymptomatic. The severity of symptoms is most dependent on the ventricular rate; the more rapid the ventricular rate the more likely the patient will have symptoms. The main clinical issue with atrial fibrillation is increased risk of stroke. Since the atria are not contracting normally, blood pooling on the left atrium can facilitate development of blood clots. If the blood clot travels (embolizes) to the brain, blood supply to a part of the brain is lost, and a stroke develops.

Irregular Narrow QRS tachycardia

Atrial fibrillation (initiation)

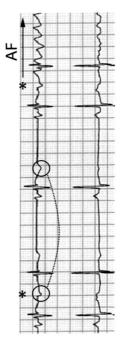

Figure 11.4:
Initiation of atrial fibrillation. In this case premature atrial contractions (*) are either isolated or initiate atrial fibrillation. Premature atrial contractions can be identified by identifying "unexpected" deflections that are present in some but not all T waves (circles).

Irregular Narrow QRS tachycardia

Multifocal atrial tachycardia

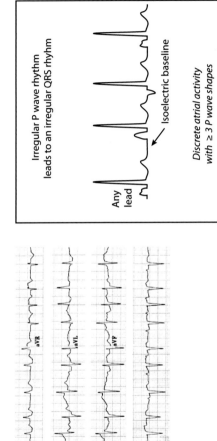

Irregular P wave rhythm
leads to an irregular QRS rhyhm

Isoelectric baseline

*Discrete atrial activity
with ≥ 3 P wave shapes*

Any
lead

Figure 11.5:

Background: Multifocal atrial tachycardia is usually observed in critically ill patients in the setting of decreased oxygen due to pneumonia or other pulmonary process or severe electrolyte disorders. It is most commonly observed in those patients with chronic obstructive lung disease.

ECG: In multifocal atrial tachycardia three or more unique sites are depolarizing the atrium at different rates. This leads to irregular P waves of different shapes separated by isoelectric periods. Since atrial depolarization is irregular, ventricular depolarization is also irregular.

Clinical Issues: In and of itself, multifocal atrial tachycardia does not require specific treatment but the underlying cause, hypoxia, acidosis or other electrolyte disorder must be determined and appropriately treated. Multifocal atrial tachycardia may progress to atrial fibrilation (where organized atrial depolarization is lost).

Regular Narrow QRS tachycardia (or irregular)

Atrial flutter

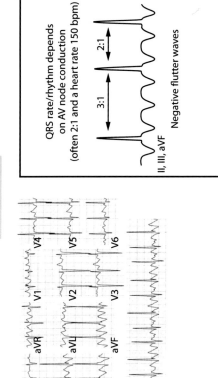

QRS rate/rhythm depends on AV node conduction (often 2:1 and a heart rate 150 bpm)

3:1

2:1

II, III, aVF

Negative flutter waves

Figure 11.6:

Background: In atrial flutter a stable reentrant circuit leads to rapid atrial activity.

ECG: The atrial activity is rapid and regular. In the most common form of atrial flutter, the reentrant circuit circles around the tricuspid valve. From our prior discussion on reentry the tricuspid valve forms an anatomic barrier that separates two "pathways." One "pathway" is formed from the narrow strip of tissue that separates the inferior *vena cava* from the tricuspid valve and the other "pathway" is simply the remaining atrial tissue. A premature atrial contraction leads to initiation of a stable reentrant circuit. Typically, depolarization of the interatrial septum and the left atrium travels from "low to high" and deeply negative flutter wavesare observed in the inferior leads. Like atrial

fibrillation, in atrial flutter there is continuous atrial depolarization, at any point in time some portion of the atria are being depolarized. For this reason, in cases of typical atrial flutter, the flatter period between the negative flutter waves actually shows a slight negative slope. Unlike atrial fibrillation, in atrial flutter depolarization of the atria occurs via a stable reentrant circuit leading that produces regular flutter waves. The ventricular rate may be regular or irregular depending on whether there is consistent conduction via the AV node.

Clinical Issues: In atrial flutter, like atrial fibrillation, treatment generally focuses on slowing AV conduction to restore a more normal ventricular t=rate and protecting against stroke with medications.

Irregular Narrow QRS tachycardia

Atrial fibrillation ("coarse")

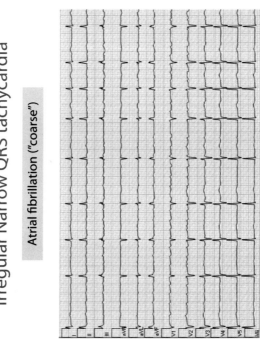

Figure 11.7:

In some cases atrial fibrillation will have periods of relatively regular activity with relatively regular waves that appear to be atrial flutter. In fact it is not uncommon for a patient to transition between periods of atrial flutter and periods of atrial fibrillation. More commonly, atrial fibrillation will become more organized for a period so that the atria are being activated in a relatively constant repetitive manner. Generally the distinction between atrial fibillation and atrial flutter is made indirectly by evaluating the QRS rhythm. In atrial flutter, although the rhythm may be irregular there are relatively few constant intervals of ventricular activation since ventricular irregularity is dependent only on changing atrioventricular conduction. In contrast in atrial fibrillation the irregular ventricular rhythm is due to both irregular atrial depolarization and varying atrioventricular conduction. This example would be classified as atrial fibrillation since although there are a few relatively fixed QRS intervals, in general the ventricular rhythm is very irregular.

Regular Narrow QRS tachycardia

Focal atrial tachycardia

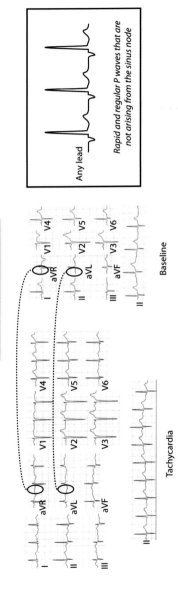

Any lead

Rapid and regular P waves that are not arising from the sinus node

Baseline

Tachycardia

Figure 11.8:

Background: Focal atrial tachycardias are relatively rare but probably account for approximately 10% of regular rapid rhythms encountered in clinical medicine.

ECG: Usually focal atrial tachycardias are nonsustained but in some cases sustained focal atrial tachycardia is observed. Focal atrial tachycardias are generally identified by a higher than expected rate and a P wave shape that suggests that the sinus node is not generating atrial depolarization. In this ECG, the patient's heart rate is approximately 120 beats per minute despite resting flat on a table. The P waves are inverted in I and aVL due to an abnormal atrial focus in the left atrium. Later when an ECG is recorded in normal sinus rhythm, a slower heart rate with a P wave with the expected shape is observed. Comparing P wave morphologies (circles) during tachycardia and during sinus rhythm is extremely helpful.

Clinical Issues: Generally atrial tachycardias are nonsustained and often no specific treatment is required. In some cases of incessant arrhythmias, medications to suppress the arrhythmia or an ablation procedure to eliminate the tachycardia site are recommended.

Regular Narrow QRS tachycardia

Focal atrial tachycardia

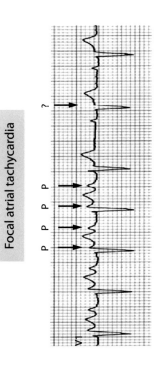

Figure 11.9:

In this example of unsustained focal atrial tachycardia, the tachycardia terminates and allows comparison between atrial tachycardia and sinus rhythm in the same strip. If the rate of the focal atrial tachycardia is fast enough, not every atrial depolarization will conduct to the ventricles to produce a QRS complex. Remember this represents normal AV node function and does not imply AV nodal disease. Blocked atrial depolarization that did not conduct to the ventricles.

P waves can be identified by comparing the QRS complex and T waves during tachycardia with the QRS and T wave during sinus rhythm. In this case a deflection in the terminal portion of the QRS during tachycardia is not observed during sinus rhythm (?) and must have represented atrial depolarization that did not conduct to the ventricles.

Regular Narrow QRS tachycardia

AV node reentrant tachycardia (AVNRT)

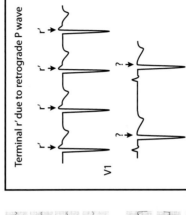

Terminal r' due to retrograde P wave

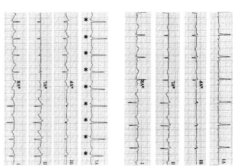

Figure 11.10:

Background: AV node reentrant tachycardia (often called AVNRT) is the most common cause of rapid regular heart rates in young adults. It is more common in women than men.

ECG: In AV node reentrant tachycardia, a reentrant circuit within the AV node and adjacent tissue leads to a rapid narrow complex tachycardia. The rapid activity from the AV node leads to retrograde activation of the atria and almost simultaneous activation of the ventricles. The P wave is often obscured but may be seen as a small r' wave in lead V₁. It is extremely useful to compare the ECG in tachycardia to the ECG in sinus rhythm. In this example the top four rows show the ECG during tachycardia and the bottom four rows show the ECG during sinus rhythm after the tachycardia has resolved. The retrograde P wave (*) can be seen slightly after the QRS complex.

Clinical Issues: AVNRT is not associated with life threatening problems, but if the episodes of tachycardia are frequent enough can lead to significant reduction in quality of life. Emergently, AVNRT is treated with intravenous adenosine that will often terminate the reentrant loop by causing transient block within the AV node.

Regular Narrow QRS tachycardia

Automatic junctional tachycardia

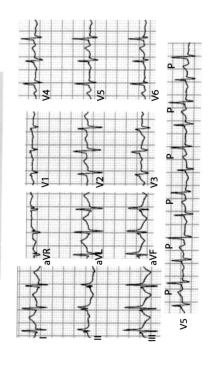

Figure 11.11:

Background: The spontaneous depolarization rate of the AV node is 35–50bpm. A much rarer cause of tachycardia from the AV nodal region is increased automaticity.

ECG: Increased automaticity from the AV node results in a narrow complex tachycardia that is not preceded by P waves. By ECG it is impossible to differentiate between increased automaticity and reentry from the AV node. However, automatic junctional tachycardia is more commonly associated with retrograde atrial block. When retrograde block is present there are fewer P waves than QRS complexes. In this example P waves can be seen between some but not all the QRS complexes.

Clinical Issues: Increased automaticity of the AV node can be seen in two very different conditions. In newborns rapid automaticity from the AV node can be observed. It is often transient, but in some cases, particularly if it is associated with other heart abnormalities, it will continue and require drug treatment. In adults that have undergone cardiac surgery, transient automaticity from the AV node may develop but rarely requires treatment.

Regular Narrow QRS tachycardia

Atrioventricular reentrant tachycardia (AVRT)

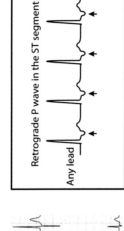

Retrograde P wave in the ST segment

Any lead

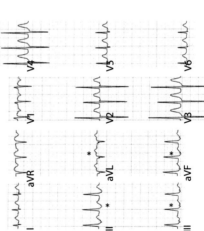

Figure 11.12:

Background: Atrioventricular reentrant tachycardia (AVRT) due to an accessory pathway is the second most common cause of episodes of rapid regular heart rates in young adults (after AVNRT).

ECG: An accessory pathway can be involved in several different tachycardias. In the most common form, a reentrant circuit develops where the AV node and His bundle depolarize the ventricles and the atria are depolarized by the accessory pathway. This leads to a narrow complex tachycardia, that is often called orthodromic reciprocating tachycardia or ORT because the AV node is activated normally ("ortho") and the atria and ventricles are depolarized in a "back and forth" or reciprocating fashion. Since the atria are depolarized after the ventricles, the P wave is usually seen in the ST segment.

Clinical Issues: Emergently, almost any regular tachycardia is treated with adenosine. Adenosine will usually terminate AVNRT or AVRT by blocking conduction in the AV node, which will suddenly stop the reentrant circuit. Sometimes there is confusion on whether adenosine can be used safely in the setting of an accessory pathway because of concern about more rapid activation of the ventricles via the accessory pathway. Remember this is a concern only if the patient has atrial fibrillation or flutter and the ventricles are activated both via the accessory pathway and the AV node (Figures 11.1 and 11.29). This condition leads to a rapid irregular tachycardia with a wide QRS complex. In ORT, since the accessory pathway is conducting "backwards" and activating the atria in a regular fashion, adenosine will usually terminate the tachycardia without any problems.

Regular Narrow QRS tachycardia

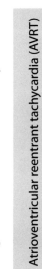

Atrioventricular reentrant tachycardia (AVRT)

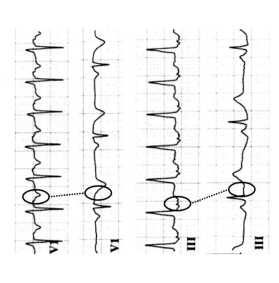

Figure 11.13:

In any patient with a supraventricular tachycardia, comparing an ECG during tachycardia and sinus rhythm is extremely useful. The location of the P wave during tachycardia can be more easily identified by carefully identifying any differences in the QRS, ST segment, or T wave (circles). In this patient with an accessory pathway, notice that the baseline QRS during sinus rhythm has a normal PR interval and no delta wave (Chapter 7, Figures 7.9 and 7.10; Chapter 8,

Figure 8.3). In some cases the accessory pathway is a "one way street" rather than a "two way street." In this case, the accessory pathway can conduct retrogradely to depolarize the atria but cannot depolarize the ventricles during sinus rhythm. An accessory pathway with these properties is called "concealed" because it is only is apparent during tachycardia.

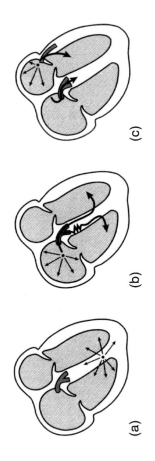

(c)

(b)

(a)

Figure 11.14:

Wide complex tachycardia may be due to ventricular tachycardia (a) or any type of supraventrcicular tachycardia in which the ventricles are depolarized abnormally. The most common form of aberrant conduction is block in one of the bundles leading to a tachycardia with right bundle branch block or left bundle branch block (b). A rarer form of abnormal ventricular depolarization is the presence of an accessory pathway (c). In this case the accessory pathway allows rapid atrial depolarization to be transmitted to the ventricles leading to a rapid wide complex (since the His Purkinje system is not used) tachycardia. Of these three choices it is important to identify ventricular tachycardia and atrial tachycardia with depolarization of the ventricles via an accessory pathway. Both of these conditons if left untreated can lead to life-threatening consequences. (Used with permission from FM Kusumoto, *Cardiovascular Pathophysiology*, Hayes Barton Press, Raleigh, NC, 2004.)

Monomorphic VT

Polymorphic VT
(Ventricular Fibrillation)

Figure 11.15:

Ventricular tachycardia (and atrial fibrillation with rapid conduction via an accessory pathway) may deteriorate to ventricular fibrillation. In ventricular tachycardia the QRS complexes, although rapid and bizarre, all have the same morphology because the ventricles are being depolarized from a single source. In ventricular fibrillation, multiple waves of ventricular depolarization are present leading to rapid and irregular ventricular activity that changes the shape of ventricular activity recorded by the ECG. Sometimes the word polymorphic ventricular tachycardia is used to describe a tachycardia that has rapid and irregular ventricular activity but with larger swings away from the baseline. For the practical purposes of our discussion, there is no difference between ventricular fibrillation and polymorphic ventricular tachycardia. Both are life-threatening and signal impending death.

"Wide QRS tachycardia"

Artifact

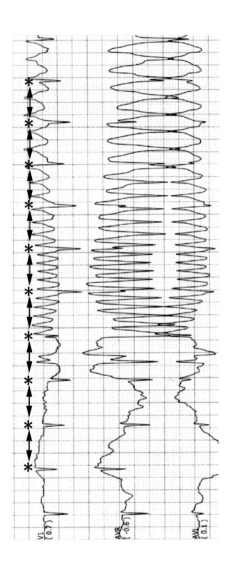

Figure 11.16:

Sometimes external sources or problems can lead to apparent wide complex tachycardia. The presence of artifact can usually be determined by identifying narrow QRS complexes (*) at constant intervals (double headed arrows) within the "wide complex tachycardia." Obviously, if the ECG changes are due to artifact the patient will not have associated symptoms. But remember the opposite statement is not true. Many wide complex arrhythmias (both ventricular tachycardia and supraventricular tachycardia with aberrant conduction) may be associated with minimal or no symptoms.

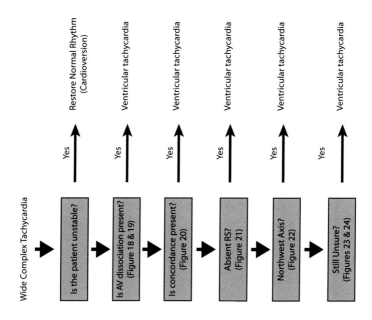

Figure 11.17:

Once it is established that a wide complex tachycardia is present, the ECG may be extremely valuable for identifying the presence of ventricular tachycardia. Again before evaluating the ECG ask "How's the patient doing?" Obviously if the rhythm is associated with significant hemodynamic compromise (low blood pressure and symptoms), it really doesn't matter what the rhythm is, normal rhythm must be restored quickly. Quick restoration of normal rhythm often requires cardioversion where a large shock is applied to the heart.

Wide QRS tachycardia

Ventricular Tachycardia (AV dissociation)

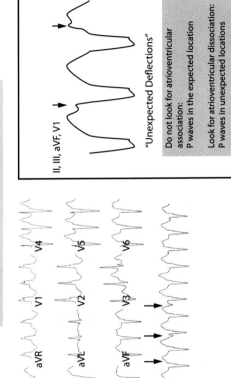

II, III, aVF, V1

"Unexpected Deflections"

Do not look for atrioventricular association:
P waves in the expected location

Look for atrioventricular dissociation:
P waves in unexpected locations

Figure 11.18:

The best way to identify ventricular tachycardia is to find evidence that atrial and ventricular activity do not depend on each other and are depolarizing independently (atrioventricular dissociation or AV dissociation). In the setting of a wide complex tachycardia, the presence of atrioventricular dissociation means that a site in the ventricles is driving cardiac activity. P waves are best identified by examining the inferior leads and lead V_1 for any "unexpected" deflections. If you think back to Figure 11.11, automatic junctional tachycardias can also cause AV dissociation, but in this case a narrow QRS tachycardia with more QRS complexes than P waves is observed.

It is important to emphasize the value of AV dissociation for the diagnosis of ventricular tachycardia. Oftentimes when evaluating the ECG, the natural response is to look for P waves in their expected location since this is how we evaluate ECGs with normal rates. However, in any tachycardia the P waves are often difficult to separate from the T waves. When confronted with a wide complex tachycardia it is best to take a "wide angle" view of the entire ECG and look for the "unexpected deflections" that represent AV dissociation and confirm the presence of ventricular tachycardia.

Wide QRS tachycardia

Ventricular Tachycardia
(AV dissociation identified by capture beats)

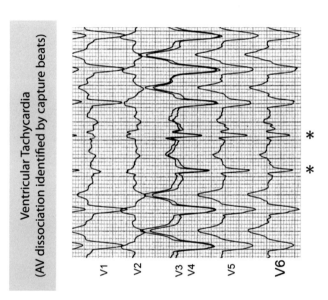

Figure 11.19:

Atrioventricular dissociation can also be identified if a QRS complex with a different shape, usually more normal appearing, is identified. This more normal QRS complex occurs because a P wave is able to conduct to the ventricles are partially depolarize the ventricles. If the beat is completely normal appearing it is called a "capture beat" and if the beat has an intermediate shape between the QRS of ventricular tachycardia and a normal QRS it is called a "fusion beat." Both capture beats and fusion beats are indirect evidence of atrioventricular dissociation and the presence of ventricular tachycardia. In this example of ventricular tachycardia, the two more normal appearing beats (*) would be called capture or fusion beats since QRS changes can be seen in V_1 and V_2. This tachycardia also has an absent RS complex in the precordial leads which is another clue that ventricular tachycardia is present (Figure 11.21).

Wide QRS tachycardia

Ventricular Tachycardia (Concordance)

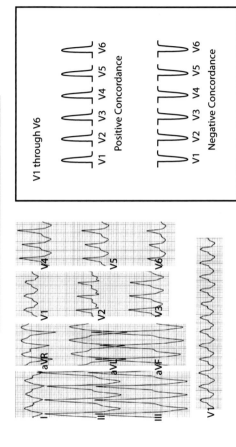

V1 through V6

V1 V2 V3 V4 V5 V6
Positive Concordance

V1 V2 V3 V4 V5 V6
Negative Concordance

Figure 11.20:

If atrioventricular dissociation cannot be identified the clinician must depend on evaluation of the QRS (collectively called morphology clues) to help identify ventricular tachycardia. One of the most useful though uncommon morphology clues is the presence of precordial concordance. In negative concordance all of the QRS complexes are negative and in positive concordance all of the QRS complexes are positive.

Wide QRS tachycardia

Ventricular Tachycardia (Absent RS)

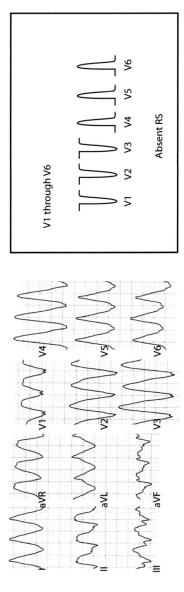

Figure 11.21:

Another useful morphology clue is the absence of an RS complex in the precordial leads. This finding is related to concordance but in this case some of the QRS complexes can be negative and some of the QRS complexes positive.

Wide QRS tachycardia

Ventricular Tachycardia ("Northwest" axis)

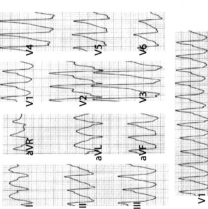

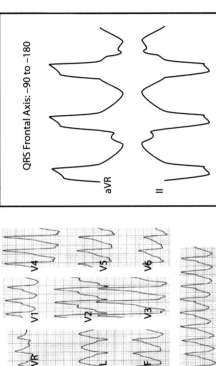

QRS Frontal Axis: −90 to −180

Figure 11.22:

Another useful morphology clue is a right superior cardiac axis in the frontal leads, also colloquially called a "northwest" axis. As you know the cardiac axis is normally between −30° and 100°. If the QRS is between −90° and −180° then depolarization of the ventricles must be starting near the apex of the heart and it is unlikely that any form of aberrant conduction could cause initial ventricular depolarization "out there" near the tip (apex) of the heart.

Wide QRS tachycardia

Supraventricular Tachycardia (With leftt bundle branch block)

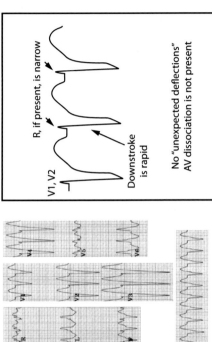

R, if present, is narrow

V1, V2

Downstroke
is rapid

No "unexpected deflections"
AV dissociation is not present

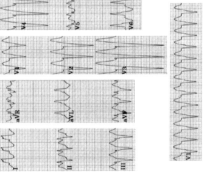

Figure 11.23:

Wide complex tachycardias are generally classified as left bundle branch block morphology if the QRS in V_1 is predominantly negative or right bundle branch block morphology if the QRS complex in V_1 is predcominantly positive (Chapter 7, Figure 7.3). Supraventricular tachycardia with left bundle branch block aberrancy is associated with a small, sharp, and thin septal R wave in V_1. In this example of AVRT with left bundle branch block aberrancy a sharp narrow septal R wave in V_1 is present. In this case it is extremely difficult to definitively say that the patient has supraventricular tachycardia with aberrancy. Whenever there is ANY doubt, treat the patient as if he or she has ventricular tachycardia. In addition, the diagnosis of AVRT cannot be made by evaluating the ECG. In this case the exact mechanism of the tachycardia was identified by an electrophsiology study (an invasive procedure that allows the best delineation of arrhythmias by using plastic coated electrodes placed directly within the chambers of the heart).

Wide QRS tachycardia

Supraventricular Tachycardia (With right bundle branch block)

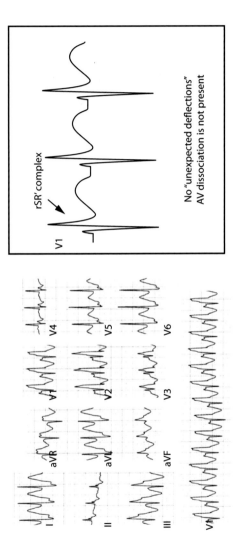

rSR' complex

V1

No "unexpected deflections"
AV dissociation is not present

I aVR V1 V4
II aVL V2 V5
III aVF V3 V6

Figure 11.24:

In a wide complex tachycardia with a right bundle branch block pattern, supraventricular tachycardia with aberrancy is more likely if the ECG has an rSR' complex with the second positive deflection (R') is larger than the first positive deflection (r). In this example of AVRT with right bundle branch block aberrancy (just like Figure 11.23, an electrophysiology study was required to make a definitive diagnosis), a large wide R' in V_1 is observed. It is worth repeating that whenever there is any doubt, it is best to assume any wide complex tachycardia is ventricular tachycardia.

Wide QRS tachycardia

Ventricular Tachycardia (Initiation)

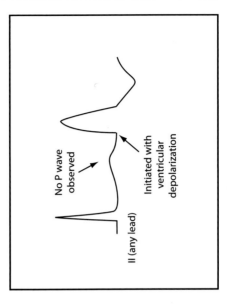

No P wave observed

Initiated with ventricular depolarization

II (any lead)

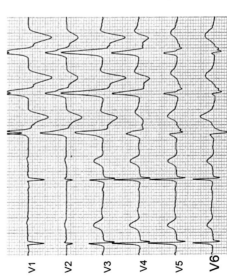

V1

V2

V3

V4

V5

V6

Figure 11.25:

In some cases, the initiation of the wide complex tachycardia is available for evaluation. Ventricular tachycardia almost always is initiated with a premature ventricular contraction.

In this example, a relatively slow ventricular tachycardia is initiated with a premature ventricular depolarization.

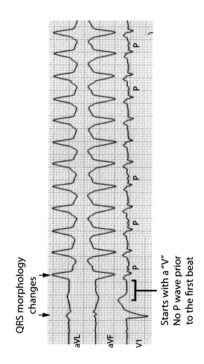

Figure 11.26:

Evaluation of a wide complex tachycardia in the setting of a preexisting bundle branch block can sometimes be difficult. In this example, the tachycardia starts with ventricular depolarization and during the tachycardia AV dissociation is present with more QRS complexes than P waves. In addition, notice that the patient has left bundle branch block morphology at baseline (the first negative QRS complex). When tachycardia starts the QRS complex has a different morphology. A wide complex tachycardia associated with a change in QRS morphology more likely represents ventricular tachycardia.

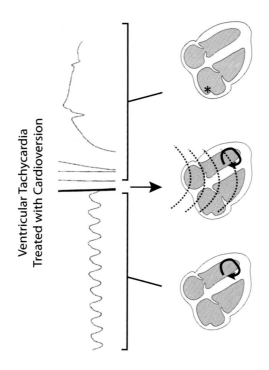

Ventricular Tachycardia
Treated with Cardioversion

Figure 11.27:

Ventricular tachycardia requires urgent treatment with medications and in many case requires delivering a large electrical current between two paddles or pads placed on the chest. This large electrical current "resets" the heart and hopefully extinguishes all waves of cardiac depolarization (both atrial and ventricular). Hopefully "when the dust clears," the patient's normal rhythm resumes. In this example a patient has ventricular tachycardia due to a reentrant circuit involving a scar from a prior myocardial infarction. Myocardial infarctions can cause patchy scarring that increases the likelihood of having the substrate for reentry (two electrically isolated parallel paths that have different electrical properties). A premature ventricular contraction acts as a "trigger" and initiates the reentrant circuit. A high voltage current is delivered across the myocardium via external pads that "resets" the heart and the sinus node begins to drive the heart (*). The sharp reader will notice that the first beat after the shock is actually from ventricular tissue with an inverted P wave in the ST segment due to retrograde conduction.

Irregular wide QRS tachycardia with a changing QRS

Torsades de Pointes

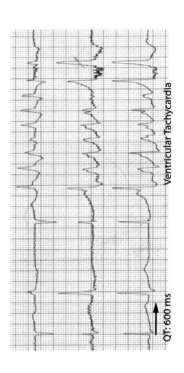

Ventricular Tachycardia

QT: 600 ms

Figure 11.28:

One special form of polymorphic ventricular tachycardia is called Torsades de Pointes ("Twisting of the Points"). In this arrhythmia, prolongation of the QT interval leads to reactivation of the heart and leads to a characteristic polymorphic ventricular tachycardia that has an undulating pattern that appears to be twisting around a central axis. Although Torsades de Pointes may terminate spontaneously it must be treated aggressively by evaluating any cause for the prolonged QT interval such as hypokalemia or drugs. In this example the patient has an extremely prolonged QT interval of 0.60 s.

Irregular wide QRS tachycardia with a changing QRS

Atrial fibrillation and WPW (Rapid ventricular depolarizationvia the AP)

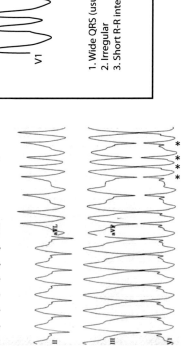

V1

1. Wide QRS (usually positive in V1)
2. Irregular
3. Short R-R intervals (Very fast)

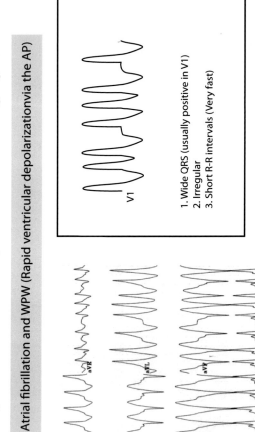

Figure 11.29:

The final major cause of a wide complex tachycardia is atrial fibrillation in the presence of an accessory pathway (Wolff Parkinson White Syndrome; Figures 11.1 and 11.14). Remember that the AV node has slow conduction properties that limit the ventricular rate if atrial fibrillation or other atrial arrhythmias develop. However, an accessory pathway allows rapid conduction so if a patient with the Wolff Parkinson White Syndrome develops atrial fibrillation very rapid ventricular rates up to 300 beats per minute can be intermittently present. The triad of an irregular very fast wide complex tachycardia should always arouse suspicion that a patient with an accessory pathway has developed atrial fibrillation. Since the ventricles are being rapidly depolarized this rhythm can deteriorate to ventricular fibrillation and must be treated urgently with either medication or cardioversion.

CHAPTER 12

Arrhythmias: Pacing

Implantable cardiac devices are now used for several different functions. Implantable cardioverter defibrillators (ICDs) are designed to automatically detect ventricular tachyarrhythmias and deliver therapy to terminate the arrhythmia by rapid pacing or by delivering a large shock. The oldest implantable cardiac device, pacemakers have been used to treat slow heart rhythms. More recently, pacing has been used to help the failing heart contract in a more normal fashion (cardiac resynchronization therapy or CRT). Most commonly, devices designed to provide CRT also have ICD capabilities. The last type of implantable cardiac device is an implantable loop recorder (ILR). The ILR is a strictly diagnostic device (it provides no therapy) and is used to evaluate patients with intermittent symptoms that are separated by longer periods of time (weeks and months). A comprehensive discussion of implanted cardiac devices is far beyond the scope of this introductory text on ECGs, but since pacemakers are so common it is important to have some basic understanding on how they function and how they affect the ECG.

Pacemakers were first developed as a way to artificially stimulate the heart in patients with bradycardia. Depending on which chamber(s) needs to be paced lead(s) are placed in the right atrium and/or right ventricle (Figure 12.1). The first pacemakers developed used a single lead placed in the right ventricle. Although ventricular pacing prevents catastrophic bradycardia, atrioventricular synchrony is not maintained. In patients with sinus node dysfunction, atrial pacing is sufficient to treat bradycardia because atrioventricular conduction is normal. Obviously, for a patient with bradycardia due to atrioventricular block, a single chamber atrial pacing would not be effective for producing ventricular depolarization. In the United States dual chamber pacemakers are the most common type

ECG Interpretation for Everyone: An On-The-Spot Guide, First Edition.
Fred Kusumoto and Pam Bernath.
© 2012 John Wiley & Sons, Ltd. Published 2012 by John Wiley & Sons, Ltd.

of pacemaker used for treating bradycardia. Although dual chamber pacemakers are more complicated, they ensure ventricular depolarization and maintain atrioventricular synchrony in patients with bradycardia due to either sinus node dysfunction or atrioventricular block.

More recently, leads have been placed in veins overlying the left ventricle to restore more normal ventricular depolarization in patients with left bundle branch block and severe heart failure.

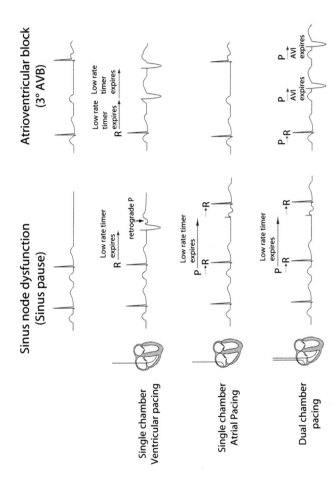

Sinus node dysfunction (Sinus pause)

Atrioventricular block (3° AVB)

Single chamber Ventricular pacing

Single chamber Atrial Pacing

Dual chamber pacing

Figure 12.1:

Different pacemaker types for the treatment of bradycardia. Single chamber ventricular pacemakers use a single lead placed in the right ventricle. Single chamber ventricular pacemakers prevent bradycardia in both sinus node dysfunction and atrioventricular block but do not maintain atrioventricular synchrony (atrial contraction followed by ventricular contraction). Single chamber ventricular pacemakers deliver a stimulus to pace the ventricles after the low rate timer expires. The low rate timer is a programmable parameter that defines the longest period of time before a pacing stimulus is delivered. Single chamber atrial pacemakers operate in the same way but with the pacing lead in the atrium. Dual chamber pacemaker can be quite complex but for the purposes of this function it is simply important to know that they have an AV interval (AVI) timer that is designed to mimic the physiologic PR interval. In this way dual chamber pacemakers are able to prevent bradycardia and maintain AV synchrony regardless of the cause of bradycardia.

Atrial pacing

Atrial pacing with "native" AV conduction

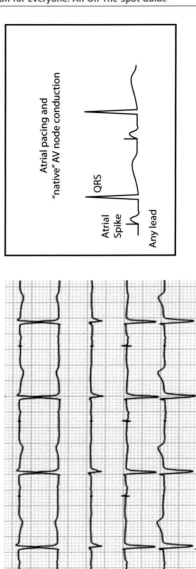

Figure 12.2:

Atrial pacing is used for patients with sinus node dysfunction. In this case the sinus node does not depolarize normally so the pacemaker is set to depolarize at a rate of 60 beats per minute. The shape of the P wave gives some idea of the location of the pacing lead. In this case the P wave is negative in aVR and biphasic in lead aVF, which suggests that the electrodes of the lead are placed in the lower portion of the right atrium. Notice in this example the patient has conduction via the AV node that produces a narrow QRS complex. However, the patient does have evidence for AV node disease because of the presence of a prolonged PR interval and first degree AV block.

Ventricular pacing

Ventricular pacing in sinus node dysfunction

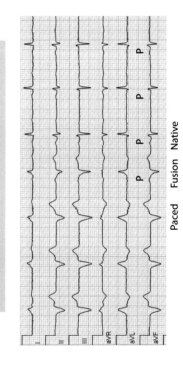

Paced   Fusion   Native

Figure 12.3:

Ventricular pacing prevents bradycardia but does not maintain atrioventricular synchrony. In this case the sinus rate is about the same as the programmed ventricular pacing rate. The first three QRS complexes are due to ventricular pacing from the inferior right ventricular apex (the QRS complexes are wide, negative in the inferior leads, and have a left bundle branch block morphology). The fifth through seventh QRS complexes are produced from native conduction due to atrial depolarization from the sinus node (upright P wave in lead II with a narrow QRS and a normal PR interval). The fourth QRS complex is due to fusion between normal AV conduction (notice the P wave before the QRS) and ventricular pacing. It has an intermediate shape that has characteristics of both the native QRS complexes and ventricular pacing.

Dual chamber pacing

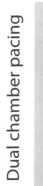

"Tracking normal sinus rhythm"

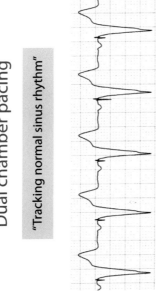

Atrial and ventricular pacing

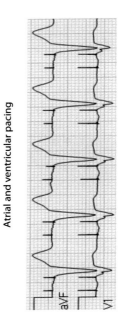

Figure 12.4:

Dual chamber pacing. Top. In this patient P waves are "sensed" by the atrial lead of a dual chamber pacemaker and "tracked." When P waves are "tracked," the P wave initiates the AV interval and a ventricular output is delivered when the AV interval expires. In this way AV synchrony is maintained. Notice in Figure 12.3 with single lead ventricular pacing, P waves do not occur before the ventricular paced beats. In the bottom strip, both atrial and ventricular pacing is present. This patient has both sinus node dysfunction and atrioventricular conduction abnormalities; we know that the PR interval is at least 0.20 seconds because no intrinsic ventricular conduction was observed after the atrial stimulus.

Biventricular pacing Cardiac resynchronization

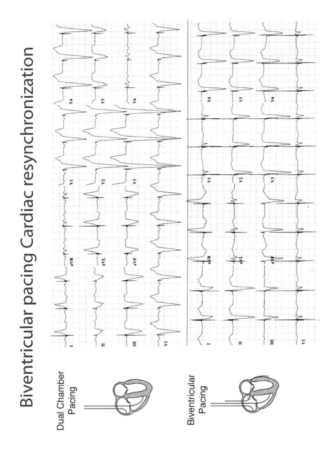

Dual Chamber
Pacing

Biventricular
Pacing

Figure 12.5:

In patients with congestive heart failure and left bundle branch block, cardiac function may be worsened because of poor timing of left ventricular contraction. In left bundle branch block the lateral left ventricular wall contracts very late relative to the septum. In an effort to provide more coordinated left ventricular contraction, specially designed leads can be placed on the lateral wall of the left ventricle through the coronary sinus and venous branches. Simultaneous pacing from the left ventricle and the right ventricle leads to more coordinated contraction. In this case the QRS is narrower during cardiac resynchronization than during pacing from the right ventricle.

CHAPTER 13

Clinical Use of the ECG: Stress Testing

Since identifying myocardial ischemia or injury is one of the most useful functions of the ECG in patients with chest pain, it is not surprising that the ECG is used as a diagnostic tool during exercise stress testing to identify patients who may have significant coronary artery lesions. The concept is simple, exercise increases metabolic demand of cardiac tissue. If blood supply is limited to a region of the heart because of significant blockages that region will become ischemic and the ECG will show signs suggestive or diagnostic of ischemia. Exercise stress testing is generally a safe procedure. However, severe complications such as myocardial infarction and death have been reported in approximately 1 / 2,500 tests. Obviously, good clinical judgment and appropriate risk stratification should be considered before ordering or performing any type of stress test.

There are several protocols used for exercise testing but all employ a gradual increase in the slope and speed of a treadmill. The Bruce Protocol is the most widely used exercise protocol. It delivers an incremental workload every three minutes. This protocol is used for patients that are able to exercise and achieve at least a speed of 2.5 to 3.4 mph on an incline of 12% to 14%. For individuals where this amount of exercise is unrealistic, several protocols that use lower workloads such as the modified Bruce Protocol, the Balke Protocol, and the Naughton Protocol have been developed. Regardless of the protocol, in general patients are asked to exercise until they have to stop due to symptoms such as chest pain, shortness of breath, or generalized fatigue (symptom limited stress test). For most protocols it is important for the patient to achieve a specific heart rate, usually 85% of the maximum predicted heart rate for age.

ECG Interpretation for Everyone: An On-The-Spot Guide, First Edition.
Fred Kusumoto and Pam Bernath.
© 2012 John Wiley & Sons, Ltd. Published 2012 by John Wiley & Sons, Ltd.

During exercise, the ECG is constantly monitored with six leads in the standard precordial positions and the limb leads placed on the trunk. The ST segment is the principal parameter monitored during an exercise test. Specially designed ECG recording systems are used that employ specialized electronics to filter extraneous noise and motion artifact from movement and also continuously measure ST segment changes from baseline.

The most common abnormal ECG finding with stress testing is ST segment depression. In order to provide some standardization for interpretation of ST segment changes, the J point (the point where the QRS ends and the ST segment starts) and the J + 80 ms (2 little boxes after the J point) are used as the specific locations of the ST segment for measurement. In addition the character of the ST segment changes are described qualitatively. There are four types of ST segment depression that can occur during cardiac stress testing:

Rapid upsloping: If the ST segment returns to normal at 0.08 sec from the J point, it is a normal response.

Slowly upsloping: The ST segment returns to baseline later than 0.08 sec after the J point and it is an equivocal ST segment response to ischemia (some patients have CAD and some do not). If it only occurs in recovery, it may be entirely normal.

Flat (horizontal) depressed ST segment: It is definitely abnormal and if it upslopes within two to four minutes in recovery, it is much less likely to be true disease.

Downsloping ST segment depression: The possibility of a positive ECG increase with the amount of downsloping and its persistence in recovery.

Several ECG findings are particularly significant if they occur during stress testing because they may signify the presence of significant lesions in multiple coronary arteries (multivessel disease):

Marked ST segment depression greater than 2 mm, especially flat or downsloping ST segment depression.

Early ST segment depression in the first three to five minutes of the test, especially when it is persistent for four to six minutes in recovery.

Severe or increasing chest pain, especially with ST segment depression.

Failure to complete at least four to six minutes of exercise.

Exercise induced hypotension.

Frequent ventricular ectopy in association with ST segment depression.

In addition to ST segment changes, the amount of exercise that an individual can perform on a stress test is extremely useful. Exercise capacity is generally quantified with METS (metabolic equivalents). A MET is a metabolic equivalent that is used to quantify cardiovascular workload and it is used to express exercise capacity. One MET is equal to the uptake of 3.5 ml of oxygen/kg/min and is the average oxygen requirement from inspired air necessary to maintain life in the resting state. After adjusting for age and other risk factors, each increase in exercise capacity (METS) equates to 10% to 25% improvement in survival. Examples of the value of the METS achieved during exercise:

• 5 METS is associated with a poor prognosis in patients under 65 years.
• Failure to complete stage II (7 METS) is very concerning.
• 8.5 METS is common with a sedentary adult.
• 9 METS or more after a CABG indicates a good prognosis regardless of other responses.
• 10 METS is considered a degree of fitness.
• 14 METS is considered physically fit.
• 18–20 METS is considered to be a highly conditioned individual.
• 24 METS is considered a well-trained aerobic athlete.

The probability for ischemia and the likelihood of its severity is directly related to the amount of abnormal ST segment depression and inversely related to the slop of the ST segment. The severity of CAD is also related to the time of appearance of ischemic shifts. It is extremely difficult to evaluate ST segment changes in patients who have significant baseline ST segment abnormalities including left bundle branch block, left ventricular hypertrophy, the Wolff Parkinson White Syndrome, ventricular pacing, and digoxin therapy.

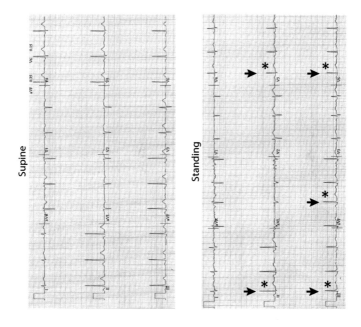

Figure 13.1:

Patients will sometimes have ECG changes simply with changes in position. In this patient standing is associated with attenuation of T waves (*) and R waves (arrows) in the inferolateral leads.

Exercise

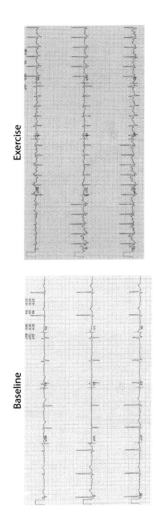

Baseline

Recovery

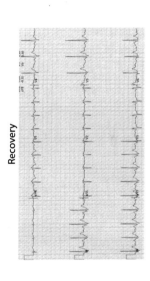

Figure 13.2:

ECG changes during a normal stress test. With exercise there is minimal upsloping ST segment depression that would not meet diagnostic criteria for ischemia. An ECG obtained immediately upon stopping exercise, shows no ST segment depression. This first ECG during recovery is critical. As noted the ECG during exercise can have significant artifact due to motion. ST segment depression associated with true myocardial ischemia is relatively long lasting and should remain in the first ECG during recovery. In this case there are no ST segment changes that meet criteria for ischemia. This stress test would be classified as normal.

Phase Name	Stage Name	Time in Stage	Speed (mph)	Grade (%)	Workload (METS)	HR (bpm)	BP (mmHg)	RPP (*100)	VE (/min)	ST Level II(mm)	Comment
PRETEST	SUPINE	13:39	0.00	0.00	1.0	68			0	0.10	
	STANDING	01:15	0.00	0.00	1.0	78			0	0.20	
EXERCISE	STAGE 1	03:00	1.70	10.00	4.6	93	100/60	93	0	-0.50	
	STAGE 2	03:00	2.50	12.00	7.0	118	102/60	120	0	-1.45	
	STAGE 3	03:00	3.40	14.00	10.1	127	120/60	152	0	-1.15	7:33 PII:13
	STAGE 4	03:00	4.20	16.00	13.4	137	140/66	191	0	-0.63	9:19 PII:16 10:38 PII:17
RECOVERY	STAGE 5	00:01	4.20	16.00	13.4	139	122/79	79	0	-0.85	
		04:27	0.00	0.00	1.0	65			0	-0.45	

ECG complex measurements (limb leads)

Lead	BASELINE EXERCISE 0:01 78 bpm	MAX ST EXERCISE 5:50 116 bpm 102/60 mmHg	PEAK EXERCISE 12:01 139 bpm	TEST END RECOVERY 4:00 69 bpm 122/79 mmHg
I	0.10 mm -0.07 m/Vs	-0.25 -0.44	0.25 1.00	0.00 -0.01
II	0.20 -0.23	-1.55 -0.12	-0.85 1.88	-0.60 0.46
III	0.05 0.01	-1.25 -0.35	-1.05 0.67	-0.60 0.28
aVR	-0.15 -0.41	0.85 -0.81	0.30 1.69	0.30 0.47
aVL	0.00 -0.56	0.45 -0.51	0.65 0.00	0.25 -0.41
aVF	0.10 -0.10	-1.40 -0.11	-0.95 1.25	-0.55 0.41

ECG complex measurements (precordial leads)

Lead	BASELINE EXERCISE 0:01 78 bpm	MAX ST EXERCISE 5:50 116 bpm 102/60 mmHg	PEAK EXERCISE 12:01 139 bpm	TEST END RECOVERY 4:00 69 bpm 122/79 mmHg
V1	-0.05 -0.32	0.25 -0.90	-0.10 -0.90	0.25 -0.38
V2	0.05 -0.32	0.45 -0.57	0.25 -0.41	0.25 -0.44
V3	-0.05 -0.12	1.10 0.01	-0.75 0.71	0.45 0.04
V4	0.10 -0.19	1.30 0.35	-0.75 1.30	-0.50 0.16
V5	0.15 -0.01	-1.15 0.28	-0.89 1.30	-0.40 0.32
V6	0.20 0.07	-0.90 0.27	-0.55 1.31	-0.30 0.11

Figure 13.3:

All commercially available machines used for stress testing will provide a summary of results. The format of the summary will vary from hospital to hospital. In this case, two summary sheets from the patient in Figure 13.2 are shown.

Top: In this example, the first summary sheet shows exercise time, conditions (speed and grade), achieved workload in METS, hemodynamic measurements – HR: heart rate, BP: blood pressure; RRP: rate pressure product (heart rate multiplied by the peak systolic blood pressure at a given point in the study); and ST: segment changes.

Bottom: Representative ECG recordings at critical times for all 12 leads are shown. Absolute values for J point change

and the relative change of the j+80 ms point for each lead are calculated by the computer from stored digital tracings and displayed. In this example ST segment depression >1 mm is noted for leads II, III, V3–V5. Compare the computer generated tracings and estimated values of ST segment depression to the actual tracings at peak exercise and immediately after exercising in Figure 13.2. The waveforms generated by the treadmill machine through its filtering algorithms have overestimated the ST depression that was actually present. This illustrates an extremely important fact. Although the computer ECG generated summaries are useful, evaluation of the actual ECG tracings is always required.

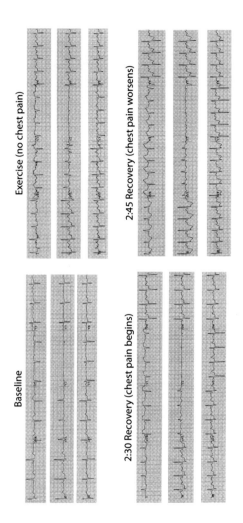

Figure 13.4:

A true positive ECG test. In this example, as the patient exercises, horizontal ST segment depression is noted during exercise. The nurse stops the test because of the magnitude of the ST segment depression (> −2 mm in II and aVF) even in the absence of chest pain. The patient stops exercising and after 2:30 in recovery the patient develops chest pain with horizontal ST segment depression in the inferolateral leads. Within 15 seconds, ST segment depression deepens and becomes downsloping. ST segment depression that is more prominent (> 2 mm), downsloping, or associated with symptoms increase the likelihood that the ECG changes are due to myocardial ischemia. It is important to note that the development of chest pain is often a relatively late event and that ST segment changes associated with ischemia are usually quite prolonged. In the bottom panel even after the pain has resolved, downsloping ST segment depression persists, particularly in lead II.

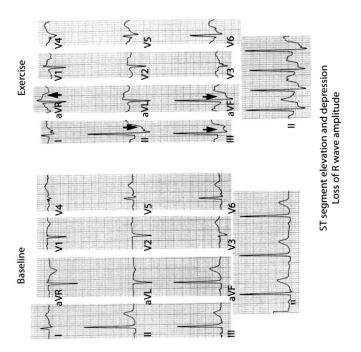

ST segment elevation and depression
Loss of R wave amplitude

Figure 13.5:

Unfortunately ST segment depression that meets criteria for ischemia can also be seen in patients without significant coronary artery disease. This is called a "false positive" because the test was "positive" (in other words, indicates ischemia) but "false" (because it was wrong). False positive ST segment depression is particularly common in women and some have questioned whether the ECG provides any value for identifying ischemia in women. To increase the ability of the stress test to identify ischemia (decrease "false negative" tests) and to reduce the likelihood that the test will incorrectly identify a patient without significant coronary artery disease (decrease "false positive" tests), additional imaging tests such as echocardiography, nuclear scanning, magnetic resonance imaging, or computed tomography are used. Patients with true flow limiting lesions will have changes in function or blood supply that can be identified by these advanced imaging techniques. In this example, prominent upsloping ST segment depression is observed in II and horizontal ST depression noted in the other inferior leads III and aVF. The patient had no associated symptoms and an accompanying echocardiogram demonstrated no abnormalities in left ventricular function. This test emphasizes the importance of symptoms for deciding whether any ECG changes are due to ischemia (rather than the other way around). This is why the importance of symptoms has been stressed throughout this book.

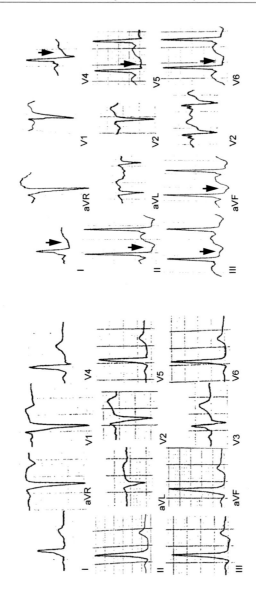

Figure 13.6:

Another situation where the ST segment depression can be observed as a false positive is in the Wolff Parkinson White Syndrome. Abnormal ventricular depolarization can lead to abnormal repolarization with stress tests. In this example the patient has a short PR interval and a widely negative QRS complex in lead V1 consistent with a right sided accessory pathway. The ST segment depression is an expected finding with stress and the ECG essentially provides no information on the presence of coronary artery lesions.

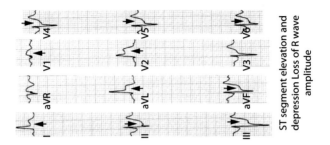

ST segment elevation and depression Loss of R wave amplitude

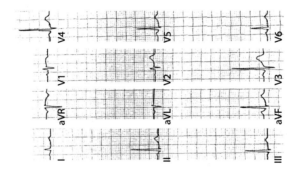

Figure 13.7:

The development of ST segment elevation during stress testing is extremely suggestive of multivessel disease. ST segment elevation is more commonly seen in patients with a prior myocardial infarction.

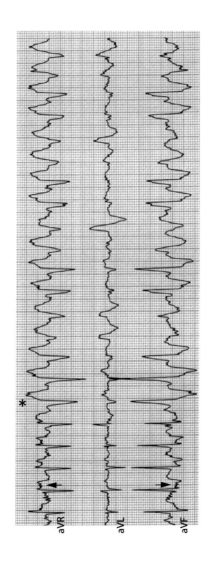

Figure 13.8:

In addition to ST segment changes, the development of ventricular arrhythmias with exercise may identify patients at higher risk of future sudden death. In this example, during exercise, horizontal ST segment depression in aVF and ST segment elevation in aVR are present. The patient develops a wide complex tachycardia (first beat marked by an asterisk) that rapidly deteriorates to a polymorphic ventricular tachycardia.

CHAPTER 14

Clinical Use of the ECG: Clinical Problems

The ECG is an extremely important diagnostic tool for patients who may have cardiac problems and for this "wrap-up" chapter it is useful to put the ECG in the context of its main clinical uses: Evaluating the patient with an ongoing arrhythmia, evaluating a patient who complains of symptoms in the past that may be due to arrhythmias (palpitations, dizziness), and evaluating a patient with chest pain or other symptoms suggestive of a cardiac problem.

Ongoing arrhythmia

In the patient with an ongoing arrhythmia, simplistically the patent has a heart rate that is too slow, a heart rate that is too fast, or a heart rate that is normal but has skips or is irregular. Now that we have reviewed the different causes of arrhythmias we can modify Chapter 9, Figure 9.1 to include the specific arrhythmias (Figure 14.1). Slow heart rates (bradycardia) are either due to sinus node dysfunction or atrioventricular block. The ECG helps identify if enough P waves are being generated and if P waves are present do they conduct normally to the ventricles.

In a patient with a rapid heart rate, the ECG is used to quantify the rate and rhythm, and perhaps most important, determine whether or not the ventricles are being depolarized normally or abnormally (Figure 14.1). If the QRS is narrow and normal appearing, the ventricles are being depolarized normally and the patient has supraventricular tachycardia. Although supraventricular tachycardia can be associated with significant symptoms, they are usually reasonably stable and generally not associated with hemodynamic collapse. In fact if the patient has a tachycardia not associated with a pulse, it suggests that some significant process other than arrhythmia is present (severe infection, severe blood loss, etc.). In

ECG Interpretation for Everyone: An On-The-Spot Guide, First Edition.
Fred Kusumoto and Pam Bernath.
© 2012 John Wiley & Sons, Ltd. Published 2012 by John Wiley & Sons, Ltd.

Arrhythmias

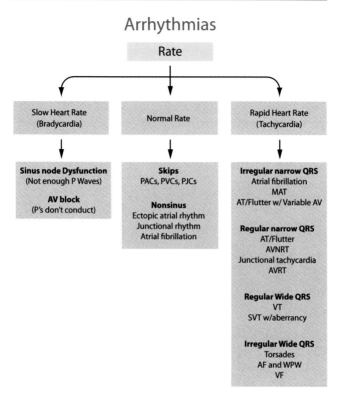

Figure 14.1:

Flow sheet for evaluation of arrhythmias. AV: atrioventricular; PAC: premature atrial contraction; PVC: premature ventricular contraction; PJC: premature junctional complex; MAT: multifocal atrial tachycardia; AT: atrial tachycardia; AVNRT: AV node reentrant tachycardia; AVRT: atrioventricular reentrant tachycardia; SVT: supraventricular tachycardia; AF: atrial fibrillation; WPW: Wolff Parkinson White Syndrome; VT: ventricular tachycardia; VF: ventricular fibrillation.

contrast, a wide complex tachycardia confirms that the heart is not being depolarized normally and the possibility of ventricular tachycardia must be the first thought that crosses the clinician's mind. Specific identification of the cause of the supraventricular tachycardia or wide complex tachycardia is covered in Chapter 11.

If the patient is complaining of an irregular heart beat, the ECG can identify whether the patient is in sinus rhythm with skips (either premature atrial contractions or premature ventricular contractions) or some other arrhythmia such as atrial fibrillation is present (Figure 14.1).

Symptoms suggestive of a prior arrhythmia: syncope or palpitations

Oftentimes patients come for evaluation of a problem they experienced in the past such as palpitations, dizziness, or syncope. Syncope is a medical term used for sudden loss of consciousness that is transient and often with a quick recovery. Syncope is extremely common and can have many causes. Generally most patients with syncope have a very good prognosis except for those patients that have syncope due to a cardiac problem, most commonly a transient arrhythmia. The ECG is an essential part of the initial evaluation of patients with syncope. The focus of the ECG is to identify patients who may have a cardiac cause of syncope (Figure 14.2). The ECG should be evaluated for depolarization abnormalities and repolarization abnormalities. Identification of an abnormal ECG makes a cardiac cause of syncope more likely.

Chest Pain

Finally, the ECG remains one of the most important diagnostic tools for evaluating the patient with symptoms that may be due to cardiac ischemia (Figure 14.3). Although this is important, remember that the patient's description of their symptoms provides the most valuable clues for the cause of chest pain. Chest pain due to ischemia is generally described as a dull pressure in the central or left chest that may radiate to the arm or jaw. The pain lasts minutes or longer (rather than sharp stabbing pain for seconds) and generally does not change with a breath or with change in position.

The hallmark ECG changes associated with myocardial ischemia, injury, or infacrtion are changes in repolarization such as ST segment elevation, ST segment depression, or T wave changes (inversion and less commonly, peaking). The ST segment elevation associated with myocardial infarction

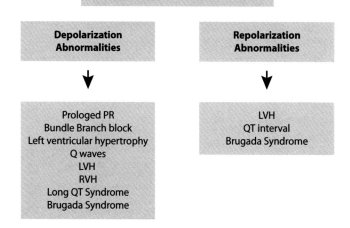

Figure 14.2:
ECG evaluation in syncope and palpitations. LVH: left ventricular hypertrophy; RVH: right ventricular hypertrophy.

is present in two contiguous leads. The presence of reciprocal changes, T wave inversion or Q waves makes myocardial infarction and injury as the likely cause for ST segment elevation. Reciprocal changes (other than depression in aVR due to pericarditis) are particularly useful if they are present. But remember that the absence of reciprocal changes does not "rule out" myocardial injury as a cause of ST segment elevation, particularly for anterior wall myocardial infarctions. In Chapter 4, only very subtle reciprocal changes in the inferior leads are observed in Figure 4.8 and no reciprocal changes are present in Figure 4.10. Reciprocal changes are much more commonly observed in inferior wall myocardial infarctions (inferior ST segment elevation; reciprocal changes most commonly observed in V_1, V_2, I, and aVL) and lateral wall myocardial infarctions (lateral ST segment elevation; reciprocal changes in the inferior leads).

The evaluation of the ECG with only ST segment depression or T wave changes can be extremely challenging. In some cases, the ECG changes

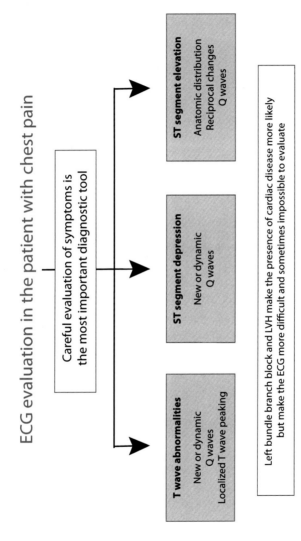

Figure 14.3:
Evaluation of the ECG in a patient complaining of chest pain.

can be extremely subtle, perhaps only present in one lead. For ST segment depression and T wave inversion, comparison with an old ECG or if the chest pain is "coming and going," associated dynamic ST segment and T wave changes should arouse suspicion for ischemia. The presence of left bundle branch block and left ventricular hypertrophy increase the likelihood that a patient has coronary artery disease or other cardiac abnormality but also make the ECG more difficult and sometimes impossible to evaluate for ischemia. Several final thoughts may help. First, more obvious ECG changes are more worrisome. The corollary of this is that for more subtle the ECG changes, either the ischemia is in a region in an area that is not "seen well" by the ECG (lateral wall), or, more likely, that the ischemia is not severe enough to be associated with large changes in repolarization or depolarization. Second, comparison ECGs, whether old or when the patient is experiencing different symptoms, may be helpful. Finally, listen to your patient and remember that symptoms always take precedence over ECG findings.

Comparing ECGs

Evaluate precordial lead placement

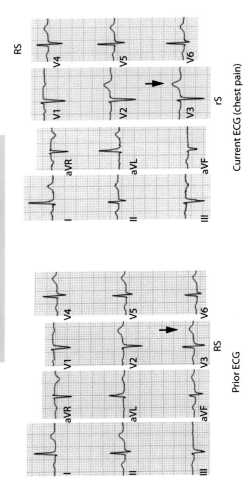

Figure 14.4:

When comparing ECGs in a patient with chest pain, it is critical to evaluate the QRS complex, particularly in the precordial leads. In this example, the T wave appears more peaked in V3 when compared to a prior ECG. However, by comparing the QRS complexes (RS rather than an rS), it is obvious that lead V3 from the prior ECG probably corresponds to lead V4 on the current ECG.

Comparing ECGs

T wave changes due to ischemia in the setting of LVH

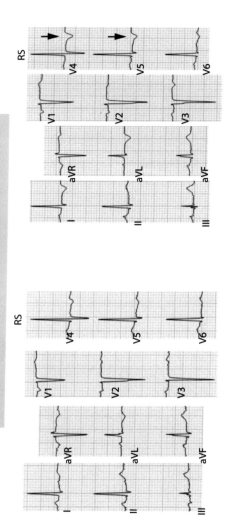

Prior ECG

Current ECG (chest pain)

Figure 14.5:

In this patient with left ventricular hypertrophy (LVH by Romilt Estes criteria with STT changes and left atrial abnormality), the ECG with chest pain is associated with more prominent anterior T wave inversion. In this case, the patient had a significant lesion in his right coronary artery.

The location of T wave abnormalities and ST segment changes usually provides very little information on the location of the myocardium at risk. The ability to compare the current ECG is very helpful in this patient who has baseline abnormalities due to left ventricular hypertrophy.

Comparing ECGs

Dynamic T wave changes due to ischemia

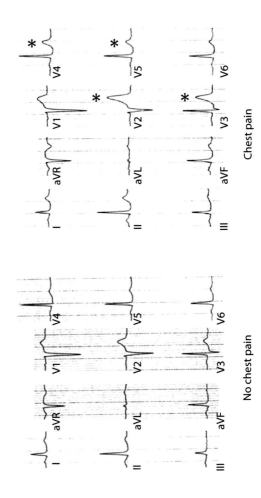

Figure 14.6:

In this patient with chest pain that is "coming and going," ECGs are obtained in the emergency department both with and without chest pain. Dynamic ECG changes associated with symptoms are extremely useful. In this case the T waves are more prominent in the anterior leads (*). This patient had a critical lesion in his left anterior descending coronary artery. T wave peaking is a T wave change that provides a clue to the anatomic location of the myocardium at risk. In this case, anterior T wave peaking due to anterior myocardial injury.

Evolution of ECG Changes in Myocardial Injury

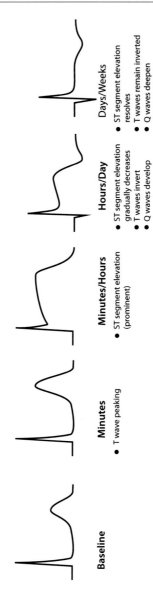

Baseline

Minutes
- T wave peaking

Minutes/Hours
- ST segment elevation (prominent)

Hours/Day
- ST segment elevation gradually decreases
- T waves invert
- Q waves develop

Days/Weeks
- ST segment elevation resolves
- T waves remain inverted
- Q waves deepen

Figure 14.7:
Evolution of ECG changes in myocardial injury. The timing and presence of these findings will depend dramatically on therapy. For example, if blood flow is quickly restored, ST segment elevation may resolve immediately or over the next several hours and Q waves might resolve or never appear.

Appendices

Additional References

Chou's Electrocardiography in Clinical Practice: Adult and Pediatric. Surawicz B, Knilans TK. Sunders, Philadelphia, PA, 2008.

Goldberger AL. *Clinical Electrocardiography: A Simplified Approach.* Mosby, Philadelphia, PA, 2006.

Kusumoto FM, *ECG Interpretation: From Pathophysiology to Clinical Application*, Springer, New York, NY, 2009.

O'Keefe JH, Hammill SC, Freed MS, Pogwizd SM. *The ECG Criteria Book.* Jones and Bartlett Publishers, Sudbury, MA, 2010.

Lists:

Causes for Abnormal Axis Deviation

Left axis deviation
- Normal variant (2–5%)
- Left anterior fascicular block
- Left ventricular hypertrophy
- Inferior wall myocardial infarction
- Primum atrial septal defect
- Hyperkalemia
- Left bundle branch block

Right axis deviation
- Normal variant
- Lead misplacement
- Left posterior fascicular block
- Right ventricular hypertrophy
- Lateral wall myocardial infarction
- Dextrocardia

ECG Interpretation for Everyone: An On-The-Spot Guide, First Edition.
Fred Kusumoto and Pam Bernath.
© 2012 John Wiley & Sons, Ltd. Published 2012 by John Wiley & Sons, Ltd.

(*Cont'd*)

- Pulmonary embolus
- Chronic obstructive lung disease
- Secundum atrial septal defect

Source: FM Kusumoto, *ECG Interpretation: From Pathophysiology to Clinical Application*, Springer, New York, NY, 2009.

Differential Diagnosis for Q Waves

Anterior
- Anterior wall myocardial infarction
- Left ventricular aneurysm
- Left ventricular hypertrophy
- Left bundle branch block
- Infiltrative Diseases (amyloid, sarcoid)
- Right sided accessory pathway
- Chronic obstructive lung disease
- Pneumothorax
- Dilated cardiomyopathy
- Intracranial hemorrhage
- Hyperkalemia
- Pacing

Inferior
- Inferior wall myocardial infarction
- Left posterior fascicular block
- Inferior accessory pathway
- Hypertrophic cardiomyopathy
- Pacing

Lateral
- Lateral wall myocardial infarction
- Left anterior fascicular block
- Left lateral accessory pathway

Source: FM Kusumoto, *ECG Interpretation: From Pathophysiology to Clinical Application*, Springer, New York, NY, 2009.

T Wave Changes and Possible Causes

Nonspecific T wave changes
- Heart disease
- Drugs
- Electrolyte abnormalities
- Hyperventilation
- Pericarditis
- Normal variant
- Left ventricular hypertrophy
- Bundle branch block
- Pancreatitits, cholecystitis, esophageal spasm
- Hypothyroid

T wave inversion
- Normal variant
- Myocardial infarction/ischemia
- Digoxin, antiarrhythmic medications
- After ventricular pacing or radiofrequency catheter ablation (cardiac memory)
- Left ventricular hypertrophy
- Bundle branch block
- Central nervous system problems

Peaked T waves
- Hyperkalemia
- Myocardial infarction/injury
- Normal variant (early repolarization)
- Intracranial hemorrhage
- Left bundle branch block
- Left ventricular hypertrophy

Source: FM Kusumoto, *ECG Interpretation: From Pathophysiology to Clinical Application*, Springer, New York, NY, 2009.

Criteria for left ventricular hypertrophy and right ventricular hypertrophy

Left Ventricular Hypertrophy	
Sokolow-Lyon	***Presence of either:***
	• R in aVL > 11 mm
	• Sum of the S in V_1 or V_2 *and* the R in V_5 or V_6 > 35 mm
Cornell	***R in aVL and S in V_3 > 28 mm (men) or > 20 mm (women)***
Estes	***Point score: ≥ 5 for left ventricular hypertrophy***
	• Amplitude: **3 pts**
	○ Largest R or S wave ≥ 20 mm in a limb lead
	○ S wave in V_1 or V_2 ≥ 30 mm
	○ R wave in V_5 or V_6 ≥ 30 mm
	• Typical STT wave "strain" pattern
	○ Without dig: **3 pts**
	○ With dig: **1 pt**
	• Left atrial enlargement: **3 pts**
	• Left axis deviation ≥ 30°: **2 pts**
	• QRS duration > 0.09 s: **1 pt**
	• Intrinsicoid deflection in V_5 or V_6 ≥ 0.05s: **1 pt**
Right Ventricular Hypertrophy	***Suggested by the presence of one or more of the following:***
	• Right axis deviation > 110°
	• R wave in V_1 ≥ 7 mm
	• S wave in V_1 < 2 mm
	• Sum of the R in V_1 and the S in V_6 > 10.5 mm
	• rsR' in V_1 with R' > 10 mm
	• Right atrial enlargement

Intrinsicoid deflection: Measurement from the beginning of the QRS complex to the peak of the R wave (less commonly called the R wave peak time)

Normal Depolarization in V1

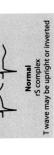

Normal
rS complex
T wave may be upright or inverted

Abnormal Positive Deflections in V1

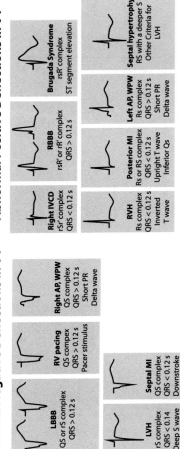

Right IVCD
rSr' complex
QRS < 0.12 s

RBBB
rsR' or rR' complex
QRS > 0.12 s

Brugada Syndrome
rsR' complex
ST segment elevation

RVH
Rs complex
QRS < 0.12 s
Inverted
T wave

Posterior MI
Rs or RS complex
QRS < 0.12 s
Upright T wave
Inferior Qs

Left AP, WPW
Rs complex
QRS > 0.12 s
Short PR
Delta wave

Septal hypertrophy
RS with a deeper S
Other Criteria for
LVH

Abnormal Negative Deflections in V1

LBBB
QS or rS complex
QRS > 0.12 s

RV pacing
QS complex
QRS > 0.12 s
Pacer stimulus

Right AP, WPW
QS complex
QRS > 0.12 s
Short PR
Delta wave

LVH
rS complex
QRS < 0.14
Deep S wave

Septal MI
QS complex
QRS < 0.12 s
Downstroke
notch

Evaluation of Supraventricular Tachycardia

1. How's the patient?
2. Irregular or regular?
3. Can you find P waves?

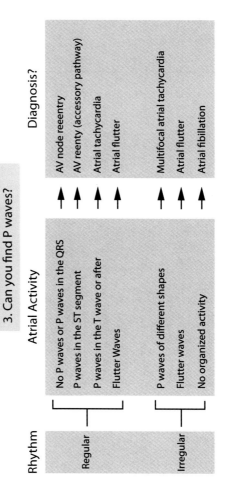

Rhythm	Atrial Activity	Diagnosis?
Regular	No P waves or P waves in the QRS	AV node reentry
	P waves in the ST segment	AV reentry (accessory pathway)
	P waves in the T wave or after	Atrial tachycardia
	Flutter Waves	Atrial flutter
Irregular	P waves of different shapes	Multifocal atrial tachycardia
	Flutter waves	Atrial flutter
	No organized activity	Atrial fibillation

Wide Complex Tachycardia Glass Beads

1. How's the patient?
2. Can you find "unexpected" deflections (P waves)?
3. "Really" abnormal QRS complexes?
   - Concordance
   - Absent RS
   - "Northwest" Axis
4. "ALWAYS assume the worst"
   (ventricular tachycardia)

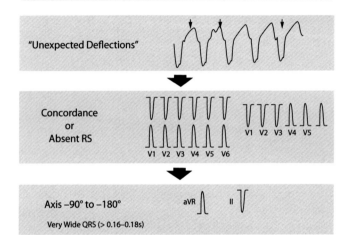

"Unexpected Deflections"

Concordance
or
Absent RS

Axis −90° to −180°

Very Wide QRS (> 0.16–0.18s)

Index

ECG Interpretation for Everyone: An On-The-Spot Guide, First Edition.
Fred Kusumoto and Pam Bernath.
© 2012 John Wiley & Sons, Ltd. Published 2012 by John Wiley & Sons, Ltd.

Printed and bound by CPI Group (UK) Ltd, Croydon, CR0 4YY

10/06/2025

14686691-0001